SEX, YOUR BODY and YOUR RELATIONSHIPS

A Woman's Guide to COSMETIC GYN and Reconstructive Pelvic Surgery

Michael Litrel, MD, FACOG, FPMRS

The names and identifying characteristics of the patients featured in this book have been changed to protect their privacy. Any resemblance to actual persons, living or dead, is purely coincidental.

The information provided in this book is designed to provide helpful information on the subjects discussed. This book is not meant to be used, nor should it be used, to diagnose or treat any medical condition. For diagnosis or treatment of any medical problem, consult your own physician. The publisher and author are not responsible for any specific health needs that may require medical supervision and are not liable for any damages or negative consequences from any treatment, action, application or preparation, to any person reading or following the information in this book. References are provided for informational purposes only and do not constitute endorsement of any websites or other sources.

Illustrations by Ann Litrel.

Published by Institute of Female Pelvic Medicine and Reconstructive Surgery, P.C.
www.vaginalhealthcenter.com

To Ann -

my life's partner
mother of my children
soulmate

Contents

Foreword

by Dr. Peahen Gandhi

Two reasons make me happy to introduce this book: One, my love of practicing medicine and my desire to advance women's health. And two, simply acknowledging Dr. Michael Litrel, a great surgeon, my mentor and my friend.

Dr Litrel's reputation is what excited me about the opportunity to work with him those many years ago. I knew that under his guidance I would become a skilled surgeon. However, it is his understanding of medicine on a spiritual level that has fueled my personal journey in making a difference in my patients' lives.

The "S-E-X" topic can be a taboo subject for many women and their doctors. Women are too embarrassed to bring it up - and many doctors don't want them to anyway.

Women might indirectly hint at their dissatisfaction in the bedroom by mentioning they are "feeling hormonal" or "too busy." Or a woman might seek reassurance while at the same time asserting, "I'm fine. I know it's an age thing." And after a comforting smile from the doctor, it's time to get dressed and wait on the pap smear result.

How do I know this? Well, I am both a woman and a gynecologist. As a woman, I have not always felt comfortable talking about sexual health with my own doctor. And as a doctor, whether I was busy screening for cancer, delivering a baby, or treating gynecologic hemorrhage, intimate health issues seemed a distant second in importance.

No doctor gets paged to the ER for an "orgasm emergency."

My own journey to becoming a pelvic reconstructive surgeon was shaped by spending years delivering babies and witnessing the pelvic floor damage that women suffer to become mothers. Surgery is not about restoring just anatomy, but also function - ALL FUNCTION - including sexuality, of course.

Why do we women rarely discuss our sexual health with a health care professional? The answer is that we have not been empowered to *change* our sexual situation. This is true whether our sexual issues stem from physical changes after childbirth or from anatomic abnormalities we are born with or even from psychological trauma.

Outdated social pressures on women to be "receivers" in intimate relationships imply that we have a passive role. Prioritizing sexual pleasure as part of sexual health has not been a focus in traditional gynecology.

Sadly, many of us just "tolerate" our bedroom role instead of embracing our intimate voices.

This book is innovative because Dr. Litrel not only prepares you with the anatomic knowledge to understand the changes in your body, but also shares the insight about allowing the healing process to occur - not just physically, but spiritually and emotionally as well.

Dr. Litrel states, "Sex is important and should be enjoyed. But true intimacy with another requires love and commitment..." Our sexual health affects our self-esteem. How we feel about ourselves impacts the health of our relationships

This book provides guidance about all aspects of your journey into achieving sexual health and rewarding relationships – whether you are trying to restore sexual function, protect your anatomy or enhance your appearance. This book is an educational resource specific to intimate health issues.

Finding the right surgeon for the job is key as it impacts the surgical outcome and ultimately long-term functioning. Dr. Litrel is THE standard when it comes to compassionate, competent and ethical care. I know you will feel empowered, supported and loved after reading this book. A surgeon's hands are not nearly as powerful as his or her heart. Helping you achieve fulfilling relationships is the *difference* we aim to make.

- Peahen Gandhi, MD, FACOG, FPMRS

PART 1

Is This You?

Considering Cosmetic GYN Surgery

In this section you will learn:

- Common problems women experience after childbirth
    - Loss of sexual sensation
    - Vaginal looseness, often with a leaky bladder
    - Uncomfortable feeling of "insides falling down"
- The two main reasons women seek Cosmetic GYN Surgery
    - Loose or sagging vagina
    - Appearance or size of labia
- Additional problems women experience but don't know can be fixed
- The 5 Types of Patients
- How your relationships can affect your decisions about your body
- What to share with your doctor at your appointment

Considering Cosmetic GYN Surgery

If you are reading this book, you are probably already thinking about having cosmetic GYN surgery. As a long-time OB-GYN and urogynecologist who specializes in cosmetic GYN and reconstructive pelvic surgery, I can tell you that you are not alone.

For example, did you know that one in three women experiences damage from childbirth that diminishes her sexual satisfaction? Physical sensation also lessens, along with a woman's confidence in the quality of her relationship with her partner.

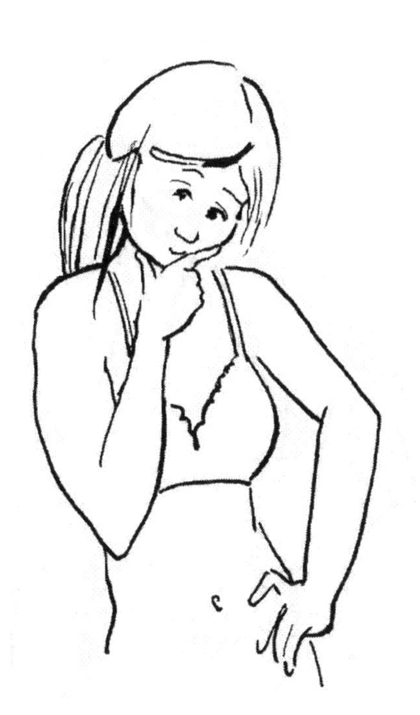

Although the vagina is designed for the delivery of a newborn, it is not possible for a baby to come out without changing the mother's body. The vagina can become so saggy that sex no longer has any feeling for her or her partner.

And it's not only women with children who suffer sexually. Among women without children, one in five are unhappy with the appearance or functionality of their genitalia. Enlarged labia (the "lips" around the vagina) can cause both physical and emotional discomfort. Extra skin gets caught during sex or in a woman's clothing. Some women may not feel physically attractive; others are embarrassed by what they see as a physical defect.

There are a number of other problems women suffer related to their pelvic anatomy or genitalia. But the bottom line is this:

It is difficult to be comfortable in a sexual relationship if you aren't comfortable with the way you look. How can you be truly intimate with another if you don't like yourself?

If any of this sounds familiar, know that you are not alone. Women everywhere suffer from these problems, often in silence.

When they finally decide they have "had enough," they arrive at my office, often traveling thousands of miles, looking for help. They want to improve their lives - what they experience with sex, how they feel about their appearance, the way their bodies function, and the quality of their relationships.

My specialty is FPMRS, Female Pelvic Medicine and Reconstructive Surgery, a medical specialty dedicated to repairing and improving the function and esthetics of women's pelvic anatomy and sexual health.

As an OB/GYN who has delivered thousands of babies, I have seen firsthand the damage women experience to their bodies in giving birth.

Now as a specialist in Female Pelvic Medicine and Reconstructive Surgery, I help women every week, from all over the country, recover their bodies, their sensation and sex lives – and I am privileged to witness the many times this process helps them heal, too, from the damaging effects of past relationships.

I've written this book to help you understand the problems you experience, why they occur, and how to think about getting help and choosing the right doctor.

Congratulations on beginning your healing journey!

You Are Not Alone!

What Women Say:

"My husband doesn't complain, but the truth is sex just isn't that fun anymore. I'm so stretched out I can hardly feel anything. And my husband can't even orgasm. I'm just afraid I'll lose him."

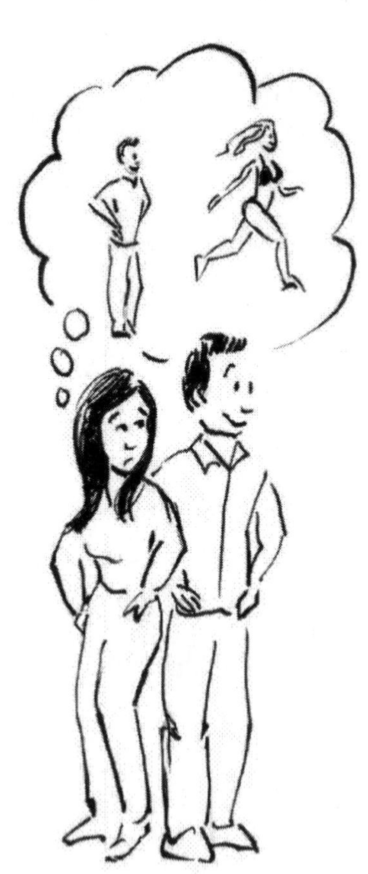

"I'm so loose I leak urine during sex. My partner was proud when I told him he was just making me 'squirt'! But I'm afraid one of these days he'll figure out the truth."

"My vagina is so stretched out my husband says sex feels to him like walking into a warm room."

"I can't stand to let him see me without clothes on. I remember how I used to look... but I'm so ugly now. How can he keep wanting me?"

"My new husband doesn't complain, but the sex isn't good. I love him, but he is a lot smaller than my ex. I am so stretched out I can hardly feel anything. I don't want to say anything, but I really want to enjoy sex again."

"I hate my labia. They are huge. And they show up even under clothes! I can't walk around in a bathing suit or wear regular workout pants. I don't want anyone to see me down there. Sometimes I feel like my labia have wrecked my life."

"I've been divorced for ten years and all that time I haven't been involved with anyone. I've just raised my kids... now I'm becoming good friends with a guy at work. But the way my body looks, I just don't think I could try taking it to the next level."

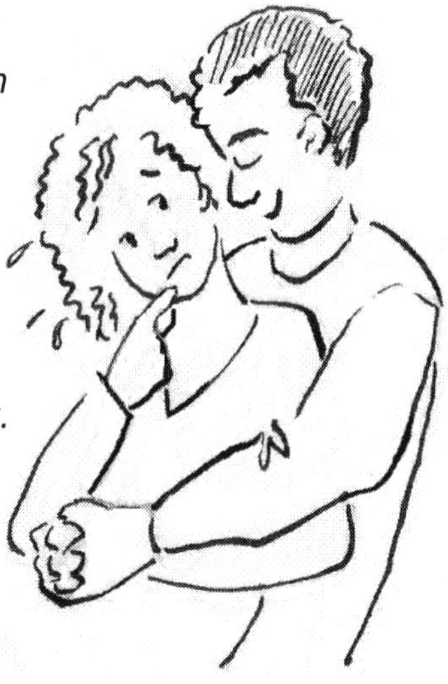

Who gets Cosmetic GYN Surgery?

Ninety percent of my patients seek cosmetic GYN surgery for one of two reasons (and sometimes both):

- Looseness of the vagina
- Appearance of the labia

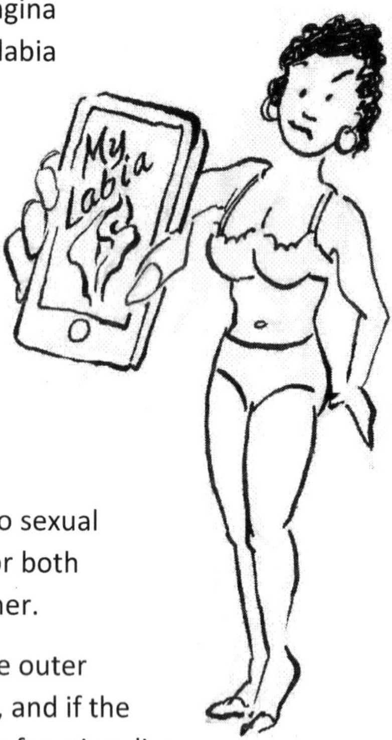

The most common surgical procedures for these conditions are, respectively:

- Vaginoplasty
- Labiaplasty

A vaginoplasty tightens the vaginal canal and the opening. This improves not only esthetics but also sexual function and sensation for both the woman and her partner.

A labiaplasty reshapes the outer skin to improve esthetics, and if the labia are large it improves functionality as well. After surgery, the labia no longer get "caught" in clothing or during sex.

Other procedures you may have read about include clitoral hood reduction, hymenoplasty, perineoplasty, and labiaplasty of the majora. And no doubt you've seen the unfortunate catch-all term, "Vaginal Rejuvenation."

The terminology is confusing. Fortunately, cosmetic and reconstructive female genital surgery is easy to understand because it's all about anatomy. You and I both can see your body and talk about the changes you want. If you do not like the way your skin sags, for example, it is easy to show you with a mirror and marking pen how your skin can be changed with surgery. If you do not like the way your vagina bulges out, I can show you with anatomy drawings what you are experiencing and how it's repaired. Some surgeries are easier, some more difficult. But in general, an anatomical problem is pretty much the same from one person to the next.

In other words, it's unlikely your problem is unique!

A Cautionary Note

As far as health is concerned, an anatomical problem that can be repaired is a good problem to have. Changing part of your body is actually simple compared to fixing common problems I hear about every day - such as feeling depressed, being overwhelmed, or simply lying awake at night with nervous worries. Addressing these feelings is fundamental to the journey of life and our spiritual health. But sadly, they cannot be repaired in the operating room – or by pills, for that matter, offered by doctors and pharmaceutical companies.

All women experience extraordinary physical and emotional challenges in life because of the loving and often sacrificial nature of womanhood. We guys have it a lot easier. It is not fair, just true. A woman spends nine months of suffering, growing new life inside her body, and then experiences the agony of giving birth.

A man spends ten minutes for his part - and then falls asleep.

So, the anatomical problems I repair with surgery are just the tip of the iceberg. Yes, you want better sex and you want to like the way you look. As a surgeon and a student of science, I will use my skill to help you get the body you desire. If you get an infection, I will use an antibiotic. If you have pain, I will provide a medication.

But nine times out of ten, you are also working on something more.

The process of life is biological - but the purpose of life is spiritual. As a healer and a person of faith, I know that real healing is about increasing your ability to love yourself and others. So much emotional pain a woman suffers is related to relationships, sexuality, and her feelings about herself.

Anatomical repair is only part of the story. Your relationships, your sense of self-esteem, and even re-kindling your joy and purpose in life, can be part of the healing journey you undertake when seeking cosmetic gynecology.

Shame Is Common.

What Women Say:

"He told me my vagina felt like mud. It has been three years since he left me, and I just haven't wanted to be in a relationship since then. I hate myself."

"I don't like the way my vaginal opening looks – it's embarrassing how big it is. I dread starting a new relationship. He may think I'm pretty, but what is he going to think when he looks at my naked body?"

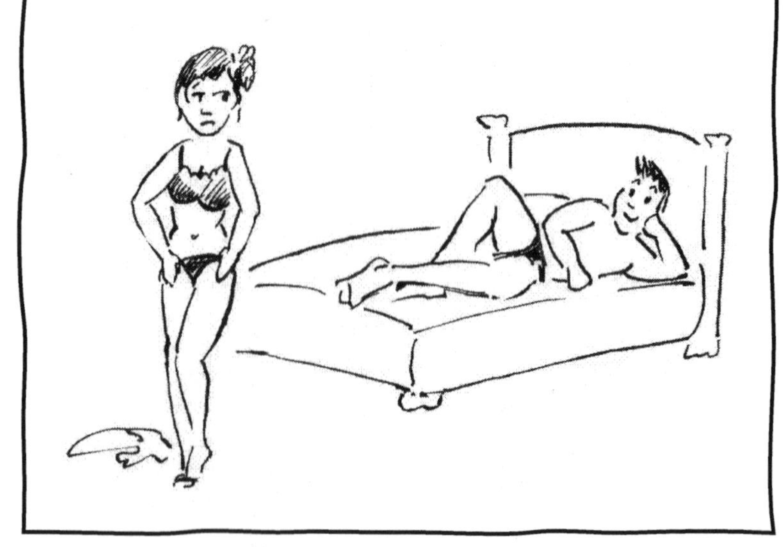

"I'm so ashamed of my body – everything feels wrong. And I have never liked sex. I just want to fix myself and move on."

"I've never been comfortable in pants – it seems like it really started when I was an adolescent. My labia got big and began to stick out so much. Last time I wore a bathing suit was ten years ago, and one side of my labia totally slipped out while I was walking around the pool - and nobody told me! When I finally noticed, I was so humiliated."

THE 5 TYPES

Patients Who Seek Cosmetic GYN Surgery – And the Reasons Why

Surgery is about repairing damage to your anatomy. I have operated on thousands of women; an operation is about fixing the body. But when it comes to restoring health, each of us is so much more than a body. Our hopes and feelings and dreams are who we really are, more than just the body we see reflected in the mirror.

Since love and relationships and sexuality are intermingled, surgical repair to improve a woman's sexuality is usually only one part of her healing journey. Removing a gallbladder does not have the same effect on a woman's spiritual and emotional life as does repairing her damaged genitalia. No one hates the way their gall bladder looks, or is sexually attracted to someone else's.

It's fortunate that fixing the body is simpler than the journey of healing the soul. Six to twelve weeks for the former - a lifetime for the latter.

So let's talk mostly about the body. But along with that comes plenty of talk about life and relationships, because those are almost always part of the picture when we're talking about surgery for sexual health and esthetics.

Most women who seek cosmetic GYN and reconstructive surgery fall into one of 5 categories – and sometimes, more than one.

Tessa Tune-Up

Type 1 – The most common patient in my office. She has children, she's in a long-term marriage or relationship. "Tessa" has classic prolapse (sagging) from delivering babies. Her vagina is stretched out. The supportive tissue around the vagina is damaged and can no longer lift her partner's penis against the nerves which give sexual pleasure. Sensation is not good for her or for her partner.

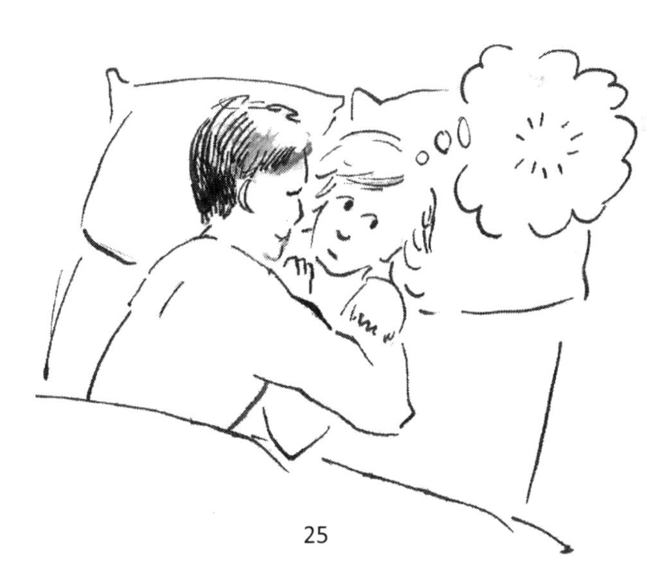

Vaginal reconstructive surgery will be the solution for Tessa.

A physical exam confirms "Tessa" has pelvic organ prolapse. Her wide-open vagina can typically accommodate four fingers without discomfort. The prolapse or sagging explains why she cannot experience sexual sensation. It also means that surgery will absolutely improve her situation.

Sometimes, Tessa has a guilty feeling that she should just "live with it," accepting her body the way it is, not looking for something better. She may believe that "it's just part of getting older." But more often, she has suffered for years without knowing her body could be repaired.

Along with vaginal looseness, Tessa may have incontinence, leaking urine when she coughs or sneezes. Prior doctors have recommended Kegel exercises. These will never hurt her, but are rarely sufficient. The problem lies more with damaged connective tissue than with muscles. The leaky bladder can be addressed surgically at the same time as the vaginal reconstruction surgery.

Lucy Lips

Type 2 – "Lucy" is the simplest type of patient to help. Her focus is on her labia or on unattractive skin around them. She often feels her labia are too large. She describes being uncomfortable in clothing, during exercise or even during sexual activity. Sometimes she has been embarrassed wearing bathing suits or tight clothing because her labia are visible. Asymmetrical labia also fall in this category.

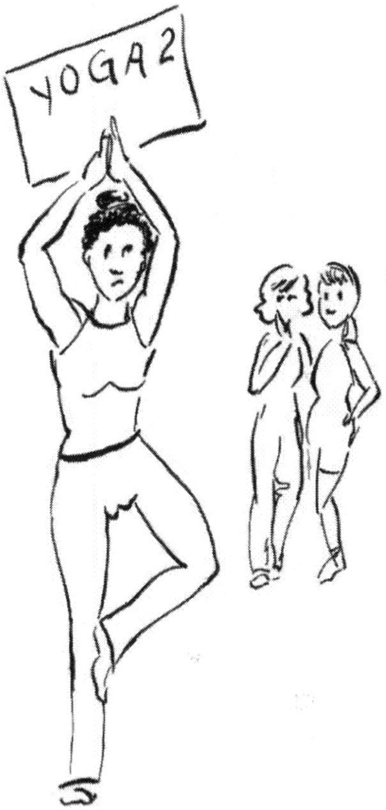

A labiaplasty is the solution.

This problem did not result from sex or childbirth but may have been exacerbated by them. Or this may just be the way her body is shaped. Although female genitalia come in all shapes and sizes, all of which are normal, "Lucy" simply does not like the way she looks or feels.

Savvy Sadie

Type 3 – "Sadie" knows her body. She is a constant self-improver, and her focus is on cosmetic improvements. Cosmetic gynecology has the added potential of improving not just the esthetics of her body, but also her sexual enjoyment. She sees her body as an asset to maintain and improve. She is value conscious in her choices and strategies. She wants to be beautiful and is willing to spend for it.

"Sadie" investigates surgeons on the internet to figure out who is best. She wants a good price but is aware from experience that sometimes easier and cheaper solutions do not work.

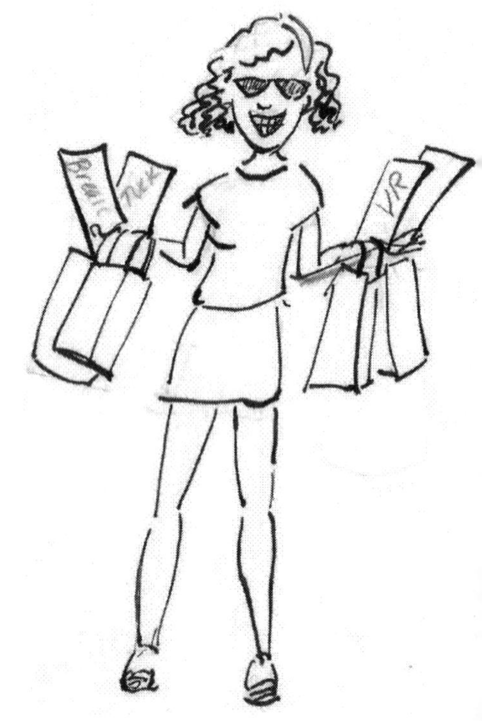

Sadie's vulnerability is a surgeon who preys on her desire for perfection with subtle criticism, prodding her to "tweak" her body again and again.

As a surgeon, I tell "Sadie" this simple truth – avoid surgery whenever you can, only do as much as is necessary, and have it done correctly.

Donna Downsize

Type 4 – "Donna" is in a new relationship, and her man has a smaller penis than her former partner. She comes to my office and says, "I love him, but..."

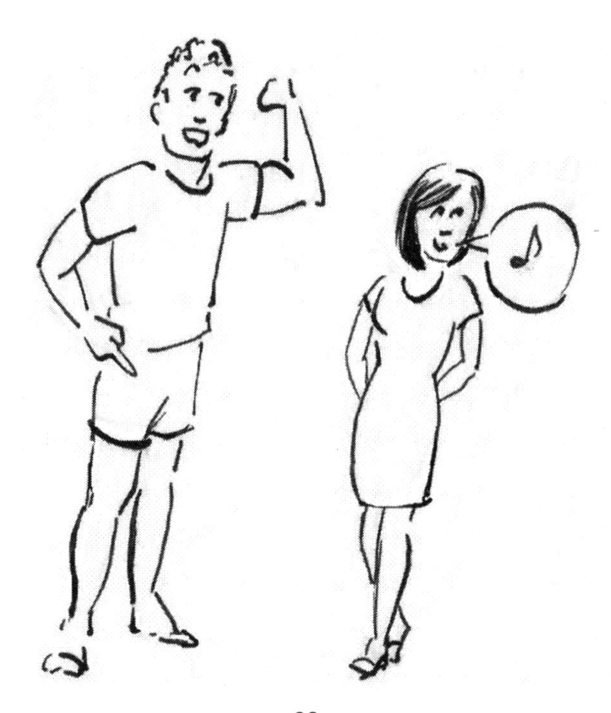

Vaginal tightening is the way to address this. As with any vaginal reconstruction, the solution is not just to make the outside opening smaller, a simple procedure called a perineoplasty. More important is tightening the entire canal of her vagina. This will provide the best sensation for sex in her new relationship.

"Donna" usually tells me that her partner is not complaining, but she notices the difference. This is important because a woman should have surgery for herself.

Della De-Tox

Type 5 – A Poison Partner or bad marriage is Della's problem: a toxic husband or boyfriend who has torn her down, abusing her emotionally or even physically. Sometimes it is just a sexual partner from her teen years, someone who said cruel things about her body that she cannot get out of her mind. She has internalized the criticism until it has become part of her. Other times she has suffered years of criticism and emotional abuse in a long-term relationship before finally coming to her senses.

When "Della" comes to me as a patient, she has typically cut the guy out of her life – or is getting ready to. She wants a fresh start. Fixing her body is a major step to get the "poison" out of her system and move on.

If Della is still in a bad marriage when she has her surgery, there is a side effect to cosmetic gynecology not listed in any textbook. It is called Divorce.

Della's healing is about breaking the cycle of an unhealthy relationship, and learning to love herself and others. It is not about seeking revenge.

That being said, the cosmic justice I sometimes see is this: "Della's" surgery might be paid for by her soon-to-be "ex."

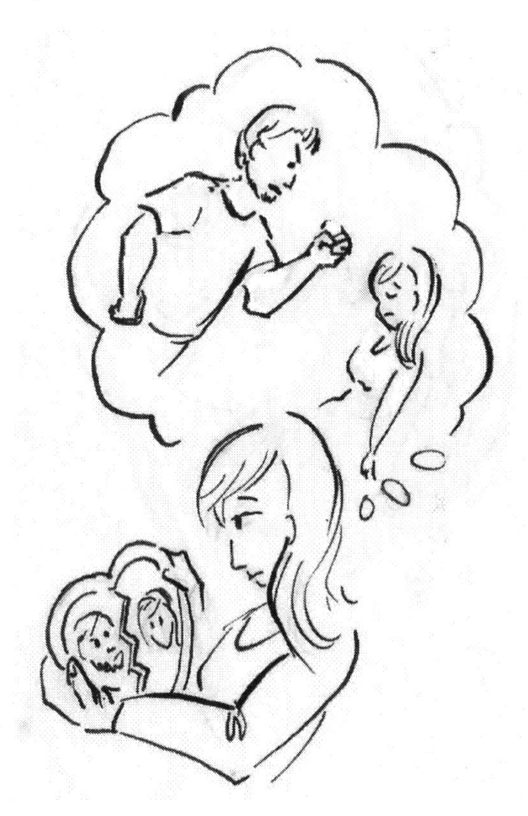

Human Beings Having Spiritual Problems

Many women have been at least a little "Type 5" in their past.

When that is the case, the healing associated with surgery is not about anatomy alone. True healing is about the whole person. A surgeon eager to operate is not what Della - or any woman - needs. Listening and understanding from the surgeon is an important part of the first step, because in this case, surgery is only a part of the healing process. What good is fixing the body if the heart remains broken? A saying I sometimes share with patients is, "We are not human beings having spiritual problems – we are spiritual beings having human problems."

Women commonly experience abuse or trauma from bad relationships. Many have unmet expectations and needs because of the selfishness of a partner, or even because of their own mistakes, which they now regret. Sexual intimacy requires trust and giving from both partners in a relationship that is loving and supportive, not just sexual. A woman's physical and spiritual health depends upon her ability to tell the difference and to make intelligent choices regarding her sexual partner.

Most women – and most men - want a stable, loving relationship. A man who cares about you as a person, not just as a sexual object, is the man who wants the best for you – rather than just the best from you. This is the man who is worthy of intimacy.

A "Toxic Partner," on the other hand, sees you primarily as a body, a receptacle into which he can masturbate. This is not someone who will support you when you need it most – during challenging life moments, in pregnancy, or in raising children together.

You can tell the difference by how he makes you feel. Listen to your heart. Do not mistake a man's sexual desire for intimacy and love when sometimes it is not.

True happiness requires loving relationships with yourself, God, and the people in your life. Cosmetic and reconstructive surgery does not lead to true happiness. But the surgery can sometimes be an important part of the healing journey.

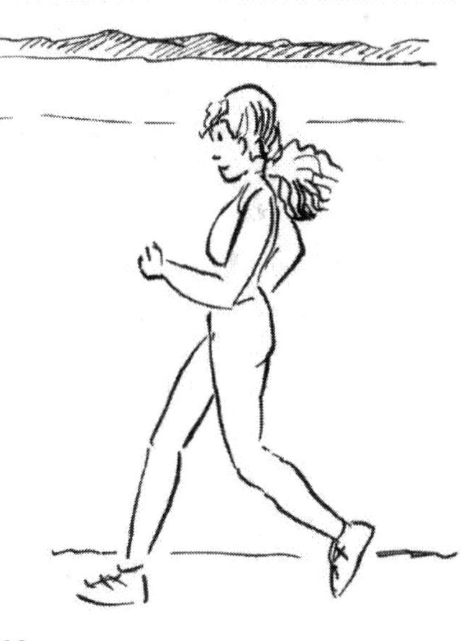

Patient Story

A Fresh Start After Divorce

"I was nervous going into Dr. Litrel's office. But Dr. Litrel and his staff were amazing. They made me feel totally comfortable, and he even had me laughing in the first five minutes.

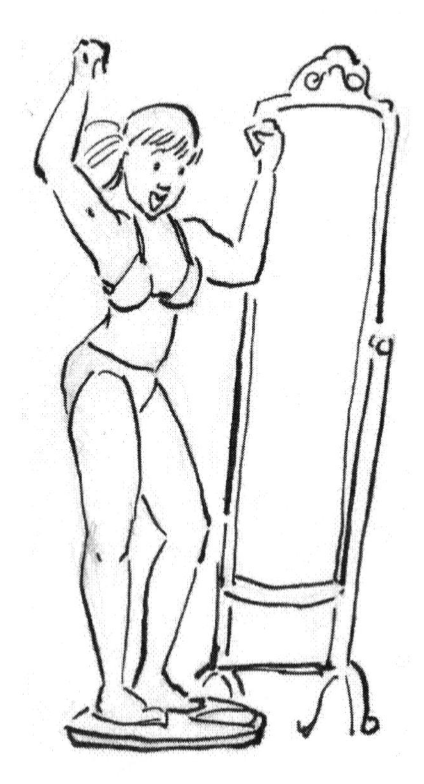

I was in a big rush to get my vagina fixed after my divorce. My ex made me feel like dirt. He got me to hate the way I look. I just wanted a totally different body.

But Dr. Litrel helped me realize it was okay to take a little time to focus on myself – just healing. And taking some time for me.

Waiting that couple months was the best thing I ever did!

I actually had the time to focus on myself, lose some weight - which I always wanted to do.

So when I went for surgery, it was totally a decision for myself. I'm so happy now - and am ready for a new relationship!"

Taking the Plunge

How You Hate Going to the Gynecologist – Count the Ways

1. First you have to wait.
2. Then you are asked personal questions.
3. Then you sit naked under a paper drape.
4. Then you feel physical discomfort.
5. Then you have to pay for it.

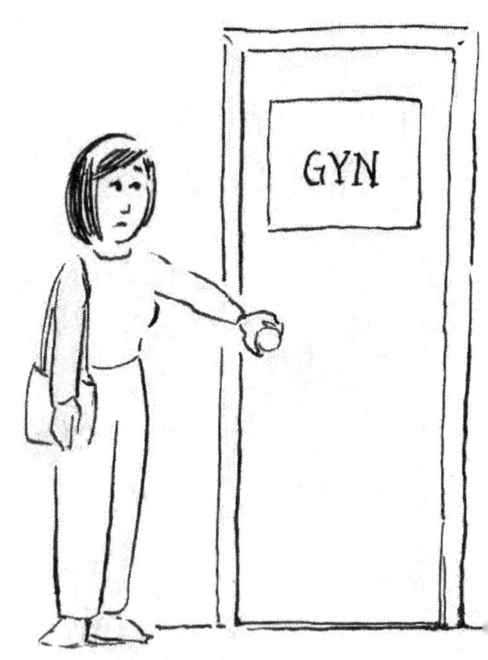

Aside from that,
what's there not to like?

Cosmetic gynecology is embarrassment on steroids. So it's no surprise it can take many years for some women to finally walk though my door.

The one thing all women who seek cosmetic gynecology share is past moments of emotional distress. Another way of saying this is that whatever experiences are driving you to seek consultation with me, we both know they are humiliating!

The good news is that I see these problems every day.

I know it is a big deal to you to talk about all this. Everyone has a unique story. But you might find it reassuring to know that the physical problems you experience are not unique. In the same way that a pregnant woman complains about swelling and back pain, a woman with vaginal laxity simply cannot feel sexual intercourse the way she once did, and a woman with enlarged labia does not like extra skin hanging down.

It is fine to be embarrassed. You will not feel that way for long. Even the most shy and embarrassed patient is soon comfortable once they come to my office. I think it is because I am not out to impress anyone – I am just straightforward, I care, and I understand how my patients feel. I treat everyone the way I would want my wife or mother treated.

It is an honor and privilege to be a doctor and surgeon. Just imagine for a moment how much God has blessed me: a patient I meet for the first time grants me a new loving relationship simply through her courage to share deep, troublesome problems. The problems I hear are those I have successfully treated thousands of times. I serve my patient and God to the best of my ability and am blessed to witness the miracle of her healing.

Do I deserve these loving relationships with my patients?

I hope so.

Patient Story

Recovering From Sexual Abuse

"My stepfather sexually abused me. I was only twelve when it started, and he didn't stop 'til I just ran away. I dropped out of high school. I slept around a lot when I was young. I just didn't know any different.

I had my first baby at eighteen. By the time I was twenty-one, I had two kids and no husband. It took me over ten years, but my life eventually turned around. I went back to school. I got a good job. Now I'm married to a good man who loves me.

But I've always had trouble loving myself. The memories hurt so much. It affected my marriage. No matter how much my husband said it was okay, I always felt dirty and damaged.

Counseling didn't help that much. So one day I just decided to fix my body. Getting a vaginoplasty was by far the best thing I ever did. Dr. Litrel really understood what was going on with me. I was so scared to meet him, but then it felt like we were just talking like friends.

I am finally myself again. I am clean. I feel beautiful. I really am. I can love my husband the way he deserves. And I feel like I can love myself, too."

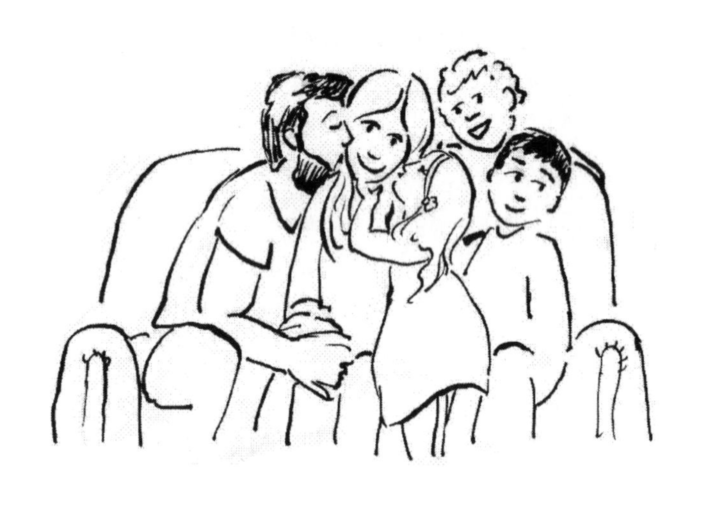

At the Appointment – Asking Questions

The basic questions I hear in the office are:

Is this normal?
What is happening down there?

The REAL Questions
... women sometimes ask themselves, but do not speak aloud:

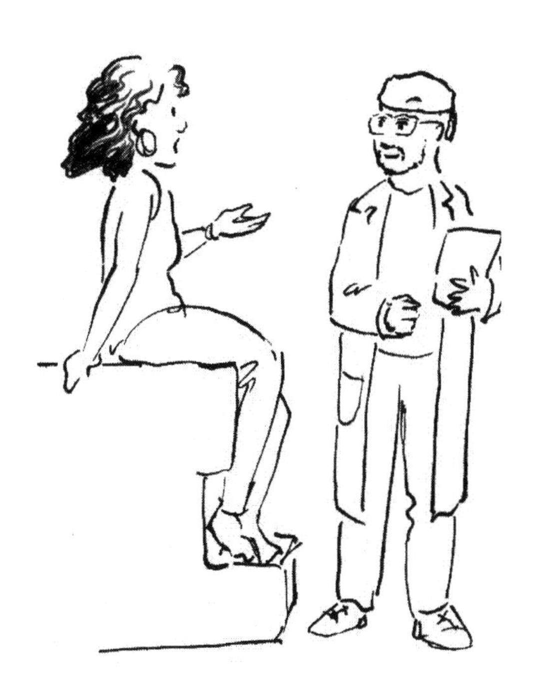

Am I ugly?

Why did my partner leave me?

Am I old?

Will my husband still love me?

Will a future partner reject me?

Will I be alone?

People go to the doctor because they are in pain. Pain can be physical or emotional or spiritual. The physical problems are the easiest ones to fix. But anatomical problems are only the tip of the iceberg.

We want to love and be loved. That is the purpose of life. Sexual intimacy is central to our most significant relationship in life. It is also the biological method by which a woman creates new life. A woman's genitalia are literally the passageway for life – and the object of the sexual attraction of another.

A woman sacrifices her body when she has children. She suffers damage that alters her sexual responsiveness, and her partner's. When the anatomy of her genitalia is not as attractive as she desires, she can experience profound self-doubt and self-hatred – which can alter her ability to love herself. This is a big problem. Loving yourself is fundamental to loving others. Love is essential to our happiness. It is the spiritual purpose for our lives.

The bottom line is that the issues addressed by cosmetic and reconstructive gynecology have many layers. The pain that drives women to search for solutions is not superficial. It takes a lot of courage to look. The good news is that anatomical issues are easy to repair.

Congratulations for taking the first step to learning more. You are deserving of happiness. I want to help you on your healing journey.

What To Share With Your Doctor

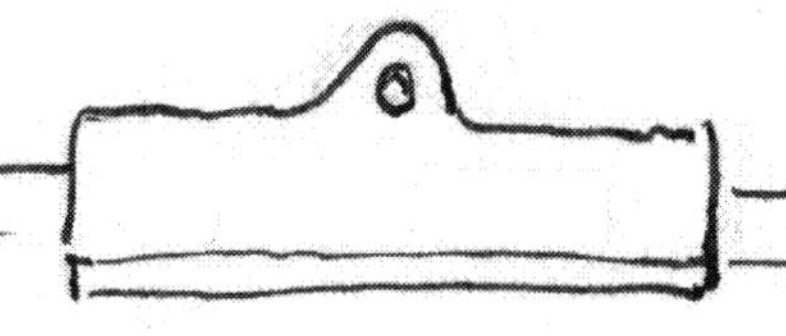

Below is some help understanding what you will be sharing at your first consultation. Finish the statements that seem to relate to you. Then share them at your appointment to help get the ball rolling.

My Body

I have almost given up on...

I worry about ...

I hate that ...

I have trouble with...

Sex

I'm afraid...

I just can't feel ...

I don't like...

I'd like to improve...

I'm afraid to ask my partner...

Relationships

I love my boyfriend but.....

My ex once said...

Pelvic Related Problems

My doctor says...

I just had a baby and now...

I notice when I cough...

Patient Story

Making It Better

"I love my second husband! He's everything I always wanted and didn't get in my first marriage. But I've had three kids – I was so stretched out that neither of us could feel sex. And I guess I didn't know there was anything I could do about it.

I put up with years of not-so-great sex - and I was afraid to say anything to my husband because I just didn't want to put attention on it.

Dr. Litrel helped me understand what could be changed with reconstructive surgery – and he helped me know what to say to my husband and how long it would take for me to heal.

The surgery was amazing. And my life has changed – I never thought sex could be this good with my husband. I am so grateful for this second chance – and that not only is he the love of my life but even the sex is great!"

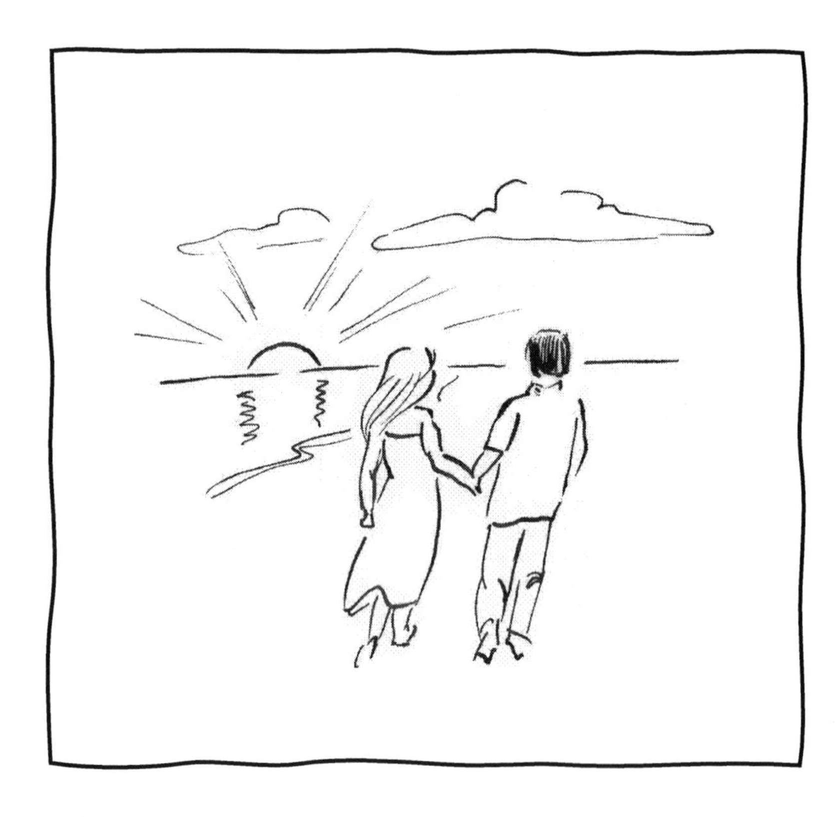

PART 2

The Basics of Sex and Your Body

In this section you will learn:

- The basic anatomy of your pelvis
    - The internal organs
    - Exterior genitalia
- The clitoris and the anatomy of sexual sensation
- How your body and your sex life is affected or even damaged by childbirth
- Why your OB can't fix it
- Pelvic Organ Prolapse – the three types and the symptoms
    - Uterus
    - Bladder
    - Rectal
- A simple physical exam for prolapse you can do yourself
- Why Kegels don't always help a leaky bladder or a loose vagina

Understanding Your Body And How Your Anatomy Affects Sex

Good sex starts with a healthy body and a good relationship.

The anatomy of the body is complicated, of course, but nothing compared to the anatomy of relationships. So we'll start by looking at the basic anatomy of your body, to help you understand the physical problems you are experiencing and how surgery can help.

The drawing on the page 51 shows the inside of your pelvis. It is a silhouette of a woman standing up facing to the right.

What Is the Pelvis?

The word “pelvis” comes from the Greek word “pellis,” which means bowl. When we hear the word “pelvis,” it has one of two meanings.

The first meaning of pelvis is, the bone that forms a big bowl shape in the area below the waist. This definition of pelvis is the one people are using when they point to the midsection of a skeleton and the bony “wings” that form the hips.

The second meaning of pelvis is not the bone, but the bowl-shaped space surrounded by the bone. This space below your waist holds three important organs we will talk about a lot in this book: the uterus, the bladder and the rectum. This second definition of pelvis is the one I will be using in this book.

Inside Your Pelvis

The Pelvic organs and their openings

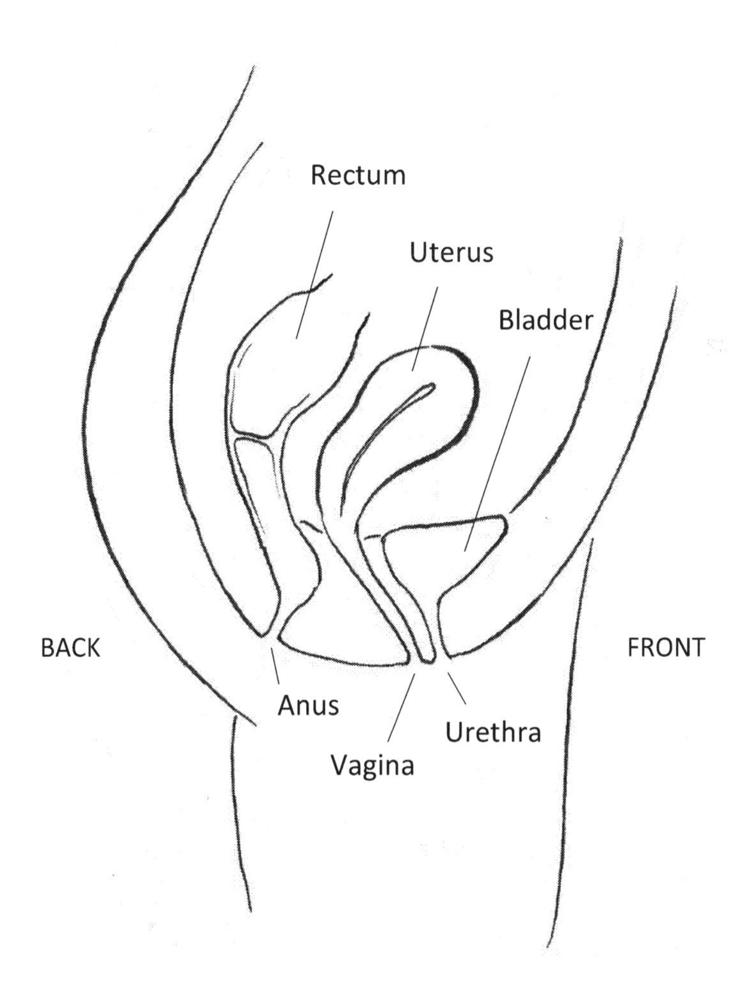

Supporting everything in the pelvis is a layer of muscles at the bottom of the pelvis known as the pelvic floor. This pelvic floor acts as a foundation underneath the pelvic organs and the structures around them.

So, what do the three pelvic organs – bladder, uterus and rectum - do?

The bladder stores urine.

The rectum stores solid waste (stool).

The uterus is where the baby grows and is the source of menstruation (blood from your period).

These three organs empty into the outside world. Urine comes through your urethra, stool from your anus, and menstruation (or a baby) through your vagina.

What Do You See?

The next drawing shows what you look like on the outside. Some women are not enthusiastic about self-inspection. But it's important to become familiar with yourself by looking with a hand mirror or cell phone camera. You may know there are some things you do not like. Understanding what you find troublesome is the first step on the journey to improvement of your anatomy.

On the Outside

Anatomy surrounding the pelvic openings

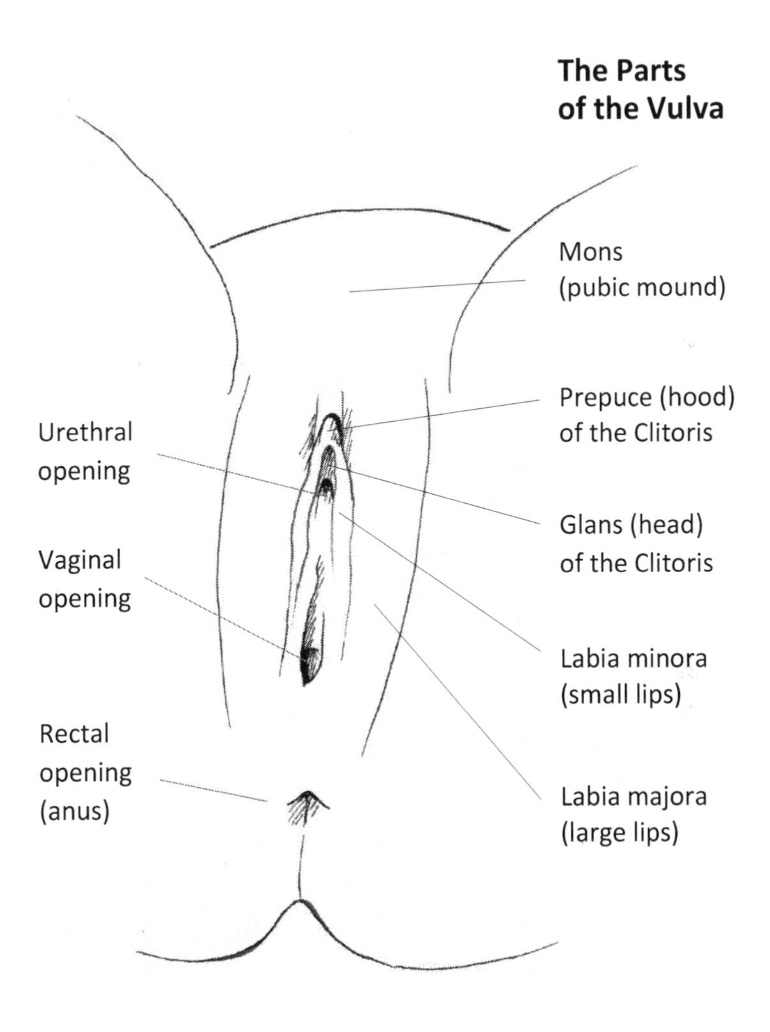

The anatomy you see on the outside is part of your perineum.

The perineum includes the entire area between your legs, inside and out. The word "peri-neum" is interesting. "Peri" means around. "Neum" means discharge. So perineum means "around-discharge." The perineum is the passageway for the body to discharge. What does the body discharge? Urine. Stool. Menstruation. And at times, a baby! The first three you simply flush down the toilet. The baby? A lifetime of love, work, and worry.

Your sexual organs are known as your genitals, or genitalia. They are an essential part of your perineum.

The genitals you see on the outside of the perineum are sometimes called the vulva. The parts of the vulva are: the labia majora, the labia minora, the clitoris, the prepuce, and the mons. Your vulva serves to protect the opening to your vagina - the fibromuscular tube that leads to your uterus or womb.

The labia majora or "large lips" are the large skin folds on the outside. The labia majora have pubic hair. The smaller inner lips are called the labia minora (small lips) and do not have hair.

Your labia majora and minora do not have that much sexual sensation. These skin folds protect your vaginal opening, while remaining flexible to allow the birth of your baby. Sometimes excess skin of your labia minor or majora may be uncomfortable or not esthetic. Fortunately, surgical correction here rarely damages sexual responsiveness. Your labia are designed to stretch during childbirth and heal afterwards, not to give you sexual pleasure. Do you want proof? You can test your labia for sensitivity to pain or for sexual responsiveness simply by squeezing or caressing them.

Your clitoris, of course, is the key sexual erogenous area. It is what feels good during sexual arousal. The head or glans of the clitoris is visible right where your labia minora meet. This is just above the opening to your vagina. Your clitoris is under a fold of skin called the prepuce or hood. Sometimes there is extra skin to the sides of your prepuce. It is commonly removed during a procedure called a clitoral hood reduction. When this is done, it is usually during a labiaplasty of the minora – a surgery to remove excess skin of the inner lips.

The mons or pubic mound is the area of your genitals you see when you stand in front of a mirror. The mons is where the labia majora or outer lips meet. If you press down on your mons, you will feel the soft layer of fat there which overlays the pubic bone underneath.

Sexual Sensation – What Makes Sex Feel Good?

You often hear that stimulating the clitoris is what helps a woman climax. You can see your clitoris where your labia minora meet under the prepuce, or hood, of the clitoris. You may have to lift the skin of the prepuce a little to see it. The clitoris enlarges during sexual arousal just like a man's penis. But even though it gets bigger, you can only see a small portion of the clitoris. The part you can see is called the "glans," the same name we use for the tip of a penis.

You might be surprised to find out that most of the clitoris is actually inside the body. This is analogous to the shaft of the penis. The whole clitoris is 5-6 inches long!

When you and your partner have sex, the movement of his penis inside your vagina can stimulate the whole clitoris – not just the part on the outside. And this is mostly what makes the friction and tightness of your vagina important for pleasure during sexual intercourse. Your entire clitoris is being stimulated, not just the glans.

Inside your vagina there is also a G-spot, distinct from the clitoris, that for some women also contributes to the pleasure of vaginal intercourse.

Anatomy of Sexual Sensation

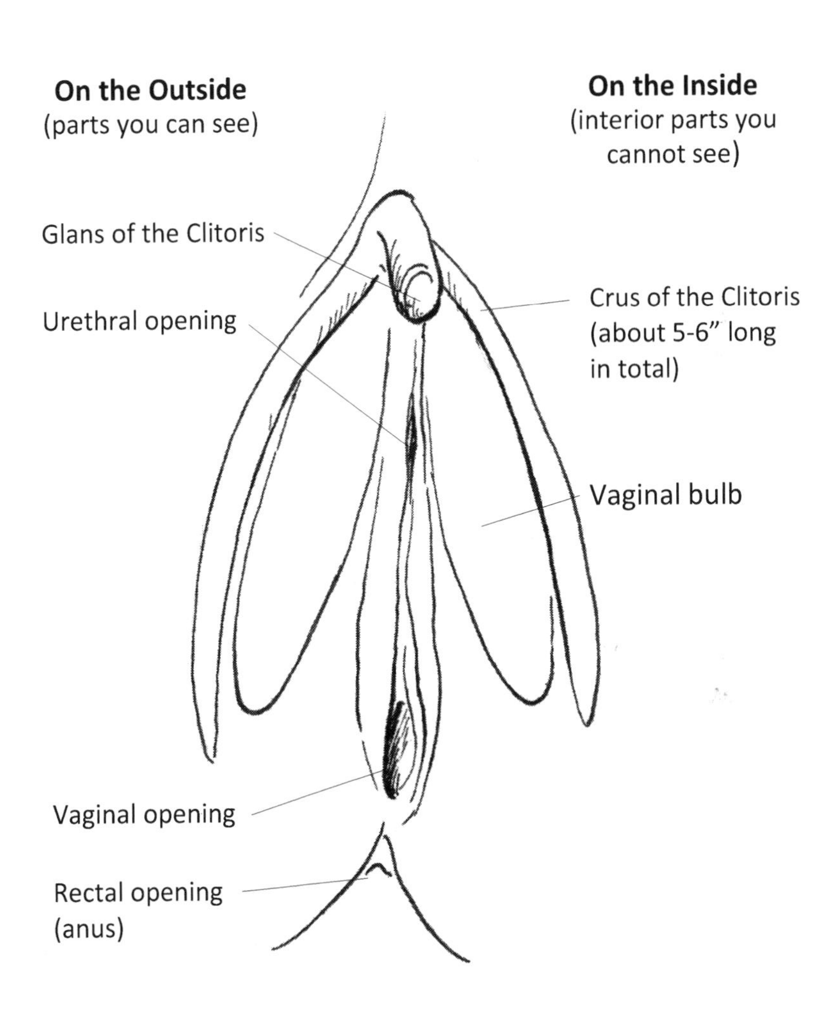

Sex was Great - and Then the Baby Came

A woman's pelvis and genitalia are designed for childbirth. But that does not mean that when the baby is birthed there is no damage. Damage to the body causes pain. Right? You close the car door on your finger. Ouch! Tears and maybe profanity. But having a baby hurts a lot more than just pinching your finger.

The comedienne Carol Burnette described it best when she said, if you want to know what labor and delivery feels like, just grab your bottom lip - and pull it over your head.

For a woman who is going into labor, I have always recommended an epidural. This is a tiny tube inserted into the spine which delivers a painkiller that numbs the lower part of the body. There are three reasons I recommend this. One, a woman's pain is largely alleviated. Two, her body is more relaxed in case of a sudden obstetrical emergency. And three, most important of all, no more screams of agony that break not only my heart but my eardrums as well.

Joking aside – parenthetically speaking, it is incomprehensible to me that some women refuse an epidural because they want the full experience of giving birth. A woman's capacity to suffer and endure is remarkable, and I suppose some women need to feel it all. I have witnessed the miracle of birth thousands of times and am still in awe of the remarkable beauty of a woman relinquishing self to give life. Her body is a literal passageway from heaven.

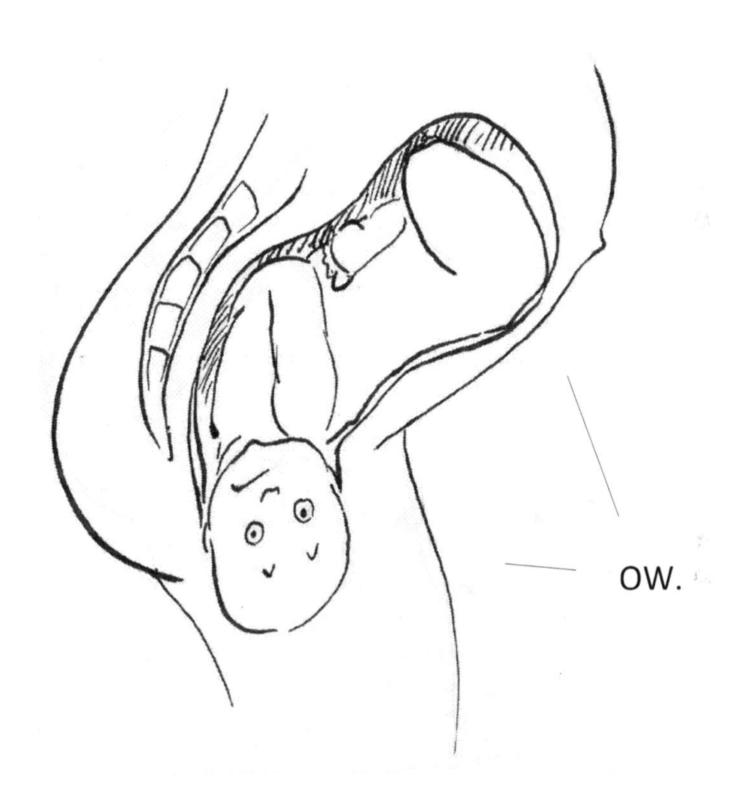

The delivery is over. There is a beautiful new human being in your life. But along with the new arrival may come some sacrifices to your body, including vaginal looseness (laxity).

Most of vaginal laxity is the result of damage to the back part of your vagina, the side closest to your backbone. This is the part of your vagina you can feel with your thumb. If you put your index finger in your vagina and press all around, you feel bone underneath your vaginal tissue. This is your pubic bone. But if you put your thumb in your vagina and press downward, you do not feel bone. Underneath your thumb is the supportive tissue of your vagina and your rectum. This is where the damage is done by the baby's head, causing the vagina to become loose.

Fortunately, the nerves of sexual arousal are generally not damaged during the birth of a baby because they are protected by the pubic bone. This is good news because you can still feel sensation even though sex does not feel the same.

Sexual sensation is decreased after childbirth, however, because the supportive tissue of your vagina no longer lifts your partner's penis against your nerves of sexual responsiveness. You do not feel sensation because your clitoris and G-spot are not being stimulated the same way anymore, not because the nerves are irreparably damaged.

Damage During Childbirth

(muscles surrounding the vaginal opening)

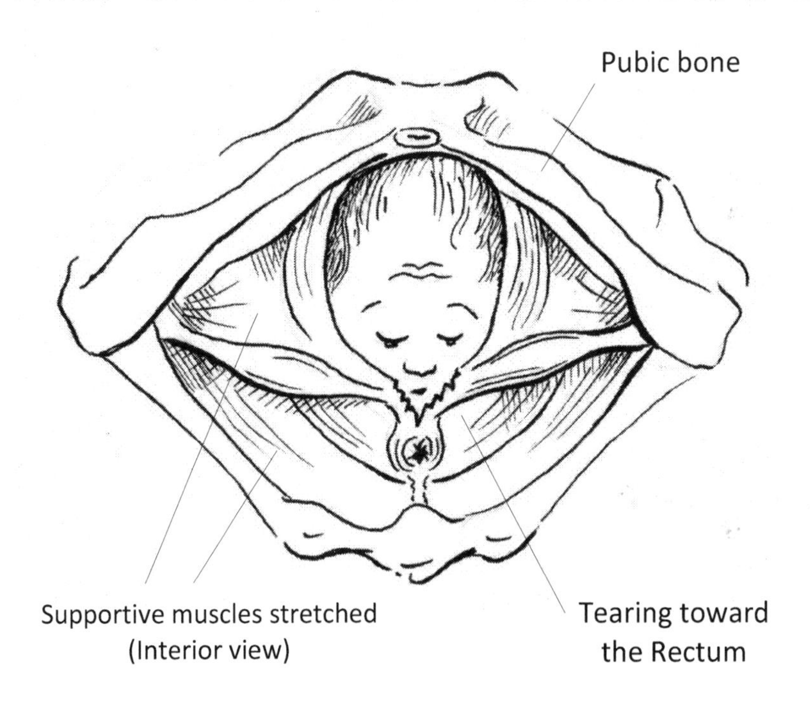

Vagina After Childbirth

(stretched and damaged tissues)

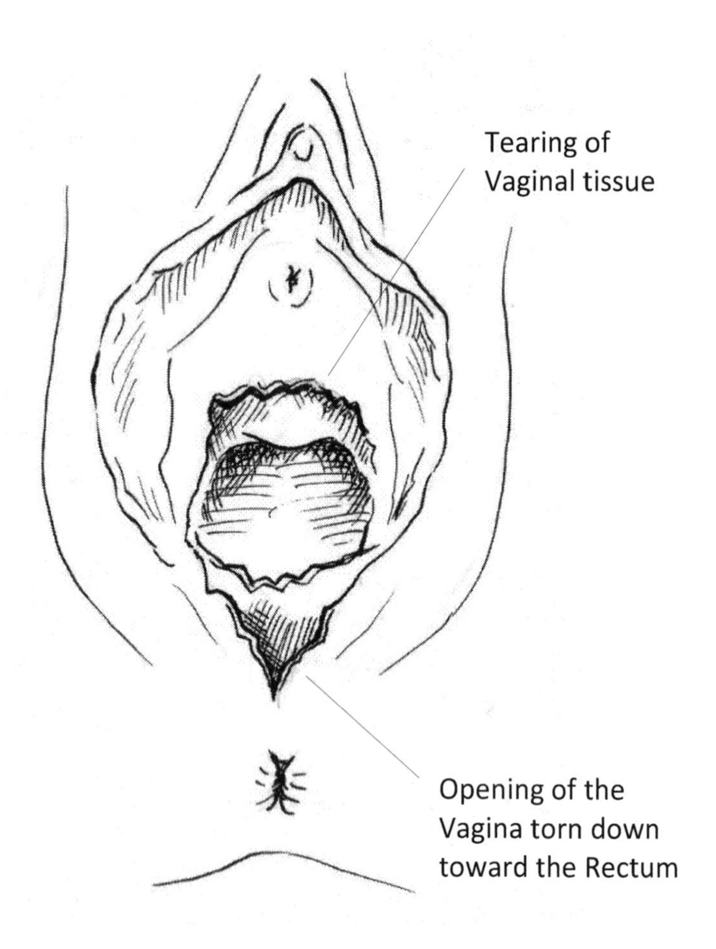

Patient Story

Taking Care of Others, Not Myself

"I noticed a difference right away after I had my first baby – 9 pounds, and I tore a lot. My doctor said to give it some time to heal. But after that, nothing on the inside felt like it was in the right place, like my whole insides had dropped and they were just pushing down. Sex wasn't good anymore. Everything was stretched and I couldn't feel much, even though my husband is not a little guy, if you know what I mean.

I waited over ten years to get it fixed. It seemed like I was always running around taking care of the kids, and my mom, who's really needy, too.

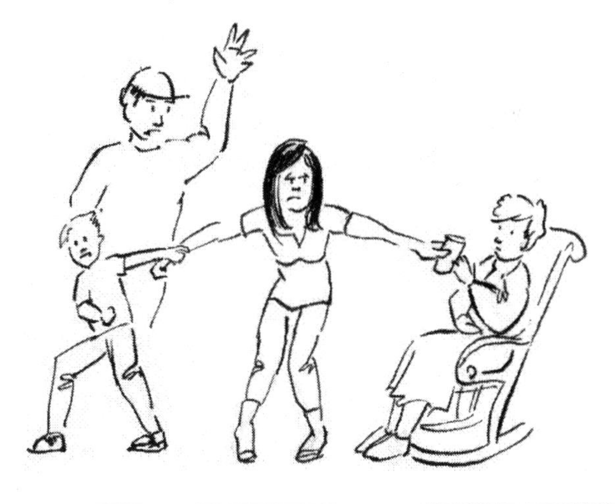

It felt selfish to focus on something like my sex life.

When I finally decided to get my vagina tightened, I came to see Dr. Litrel. He did an exam and said he could also fix that "falling" feeling! I was really excited and hopeful that something could change.

Immediately after the surgery I felt different. Everything was back in the right place – not falling down.

I wish I had done it sooner! I'm so happy I finally have my body back."

Why Not a Repair Right After the Delivery?

Why doesn't the obstetrician just fix your anatomy right after the baby comes out so you can avoid all this? You go to the doctor fifteen times during your pregnancy and spend a couple days in the hospital. Once the baby finally comes out, a repair seems the least the doctor could do.

I have delivered thousands of babies and indeed have performed many surgical repairs right after delivery. When vaginal repairs are performed immediately after childbirth, they address mainly the external anatomy – the muscles of the pelvic floor, then the layer of muscles immediately below the skin, and finally the vaginal opening. Tears in the muscles are sutured carefully together. Lacerations around the vaginal opening are repaired and the external opening of the vagina is tightened.

These kinds of repairs after a delivery used to be more common. In my instance, after my formal training at Emory University, I was blessed to have a mentor, Dr. James Cross, for the first eight years of my career.

Thirty years my senior, Dr. Cross had been delivering babies and doing vaginal reconstructive surgery since before I was born. In my first month of private practice,

Dr. Cross could stand to watch me attempt a vaginal repair for only about thirty seconds. Then he would say with a chuckle, “Let me show you how to do that, Dr. Mike.” I stood aside to watch, humbled to see how much I still had to learn. But in the coming months, I learned to repair, to suture, to reconstruct the anatomy, so that a woman’s esthetics and sexual function would not be the sacrifice after the delivery of her baby.

Over the next eight years, Dr. Cross and I performed thousands of GYN surgeries together. I was the more experienced laparoscopic surgeon, so Dr. Cross always had me do that part of any operation. (Laparoscopy is the surgical technique in which long instruments are placed through tiny incisions to operate on internal abdominal and pelvic anatomy.)

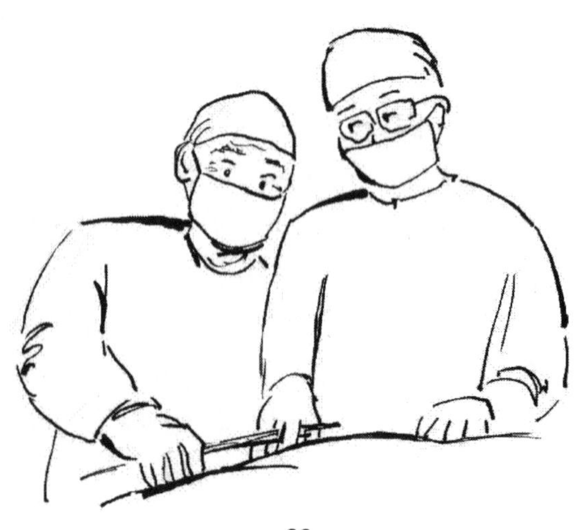

But when we did vaginal surgery (surgery done through the vagina, not through incisions in the abdomen), I simply assisted Dr. Cross. Sitting at the foot of a master, I learned how to fix damage to a woman's vagina. These surgical skills translated to my obstetrical care, so that immediately after a woman delivered her baby, I knew exactly how to fix her body so her sex life was not destroyed by this miracle of childbirth.

To be clear, these post-childbirth repairs involved the muscles of the pelvic floor and the anatomy closest to the vagina, not the deeper pelvic anatomy that is addressed with new surgical techniques for major pelvic prolapse. But my repairs made all the difference for the new mother, insuring that any pelvic prolapse would not immediately progress, and that her sexual function would be preserved, for many years to come.

Obstetrical Care Has Changed

Obstetrical care has changed over the decades. In years past, episiotomies and forceps delivery were routine during deliveries. (An episiotomy is an incision made to widen the vaginal opening for childbirth. Forceps are an instrument used to help pull out the baby's head when it becomes stuck.) These were not gentle techniques, and vaginal surgery was often necessary to correct the damage.

The trend in modern obstetrics is to no longer do episiotomies, to no longer perform forceps, but to simply perform cesarean sections any time vaginal delivery becomes difficult. There are fewer vaginal deliveries and because of that, fewer vaginal repairs.

The vagina and perineum are routinely stretched and massaged for an hour or longer to allow the baby's head to deliver without any lacerations. This is the way midwives have always delivered babies and the way doctors do now. Midwives are not surgeons, so any laceration that required surgery was something to avoid.

Expectant mothers are now taught to massage their perineum before they go into labor to reduce the chances of tearing. All this stuff really works. It's impressive to see how a large head can emerge through a small hole - with no surgical repair needed. The vulva and the vagina are designed to stretch to accommodate the birth of a baby. Massage the tissue and allow it to stretch, and it is less likely to tear.

There are many studies in the obstetrical literature that support not performing an episiotomy, and all doctors are now taught that routine episiotomy is wrong, wrong, wrong.

But just because the baby comes out with no tearing of the mother's vagina and perineum, does not mean that there will be no damage to the internal anatomy of her body. All that stretching adds to vaginal looseness down the road, no matter what anyone says. With natural childbirth, the delivery takes longer, the baby's head stretches the pelvic floor, and in the absence of surgical repair, there is more sagging and laxity later.

Because obstetricians are no longer trained in how to do vaginal surgery, you will not be fixed when you deliver your baby.

And a stretched vagina is not a tight vagina.

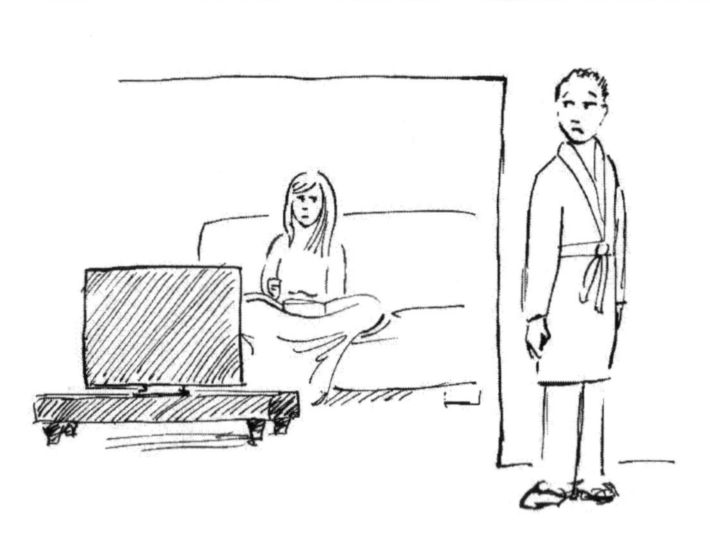

Patient Story

Why Don't I Enjoy Sex?

"I thought there must be something wrong with me, because I could never climax with my husband. I kept looking at my clitoris and wondering if it was messed up – maybe I had a 'hooded clitoris.' I am just never in the mood for sex.

I came in for an exam and Dr. Litrel asked me a lot of questions about my life… I found out I had a pretty bad prolapse – that's why I couldn't feel anything.

But he said the main problem was that I was working 50 hours a week, taking care of the kids, and my husband was doing nothing!! So he sat us both down in the office and talked to us about changing things so I wasn't so stressed out. It's really changed everything.

Now that we're getting along better, I'm so excited to get the reconstructive surgery – things should get even better between us."

FPMRS – A New Subspecialty

In 2011, a new subspecialty appeared in the field of medicine. Formally designated "Female Pelvic Medicine and Reconstructive Surgery" (FPMRS), it was formed to address pelvic organ reconstruction resulting from childbirth injuries. The first official FPMRS doctors were board-certified in 2013.

FPMRS is the subspecialty in which I am board certified.

What Is Board Certification?

Board certification is an extra step doctors undergo to gain expertise in the latest advancements in their specialty. Board certified doctors participate in ongoing assessment and training beyond what is required of their peers without board certification.

Board certified FPMRS physicians dedicate themselves to the study and treatment of problems and injuries concerning the pelvic organs in women, offering special expertise in vaginal reconstructive surgery.

FPMRS specialists complete medical school, followed by residency training in either Obstetrics and Gynecology, or Urology. To become board certified in the subspecialty FPMRS, they receive further specialized training focusing on the surgical and non-surgical medical care for the female pelvis, learning to evaluate and treat conditions that affect the female pelvic organs and the muscles and connective tissue that support the organs.

The longstanding medical specialty known as "urogynecology" has evolved or been incorporated into the subspecialty FPMRS, with the terms "urogynecology" and "FPMRS" now somewhat synonymous.

Pelvic Organ Prolapse - What Is It?

Even if a woman has a good surgical repair of the vagina and vulva right after delivery, she may still need reconstructive surgery down the road. A good surgical repair after delivery will help prevent postpartum sexual dysfunction and will delay the necessity for reconstructive surgery. But after any vaginal delivery, the organs inside the pelvis will drop down to some degree.

You push your pelvic organs outward when you push a baby out. Simple fact.

During a gynecological examination, it is easy to tell if a woman has had a vaginal birth. The anatomy of a woman who has delivered only by c-section will be not much different from that of a woman who has had no children at all. The pelvic floor muscles will be basically intact.

Every woman who has given birth vaginally will drop down to some degree. She will not, as a rule, be diagnosed with prolapse by her gynecologist until she notices the symptoms and begins to seek relief (and sometimes even then she will not receive the correct diagnosis of pelvic prolapse). A woman with prolapse might say things like, “My bottom is falling out” or “I feel like I am sagging” or “I feel pressure down there when I have my cycle” or “I wear a pad all the time because I leak.”

“Prolapse” basically means “fallen.” When it comes to pelvic prolapse, there are three places that can sag. They are the front (the bladder), the back (the rectum), or the top (the uterus).

Three Types of Pelvic Organ Prolapse

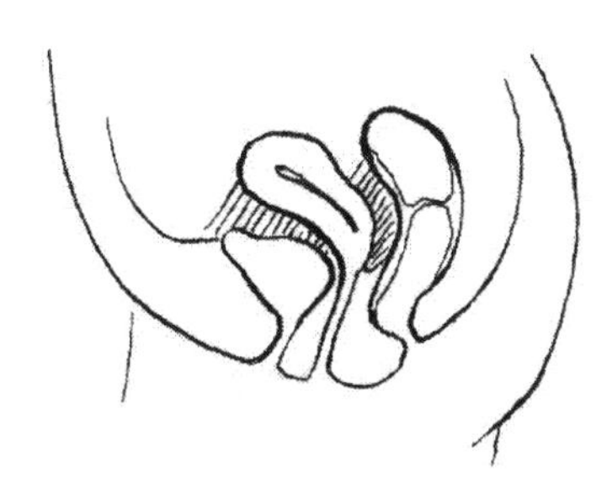

Normal Pelvic Anatomy

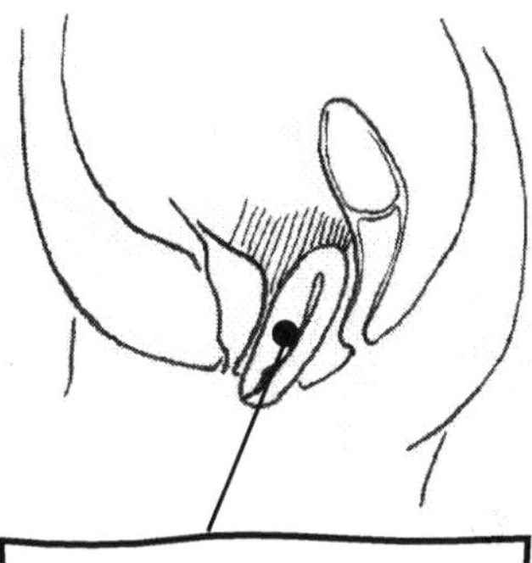

Prolapsed Uterus

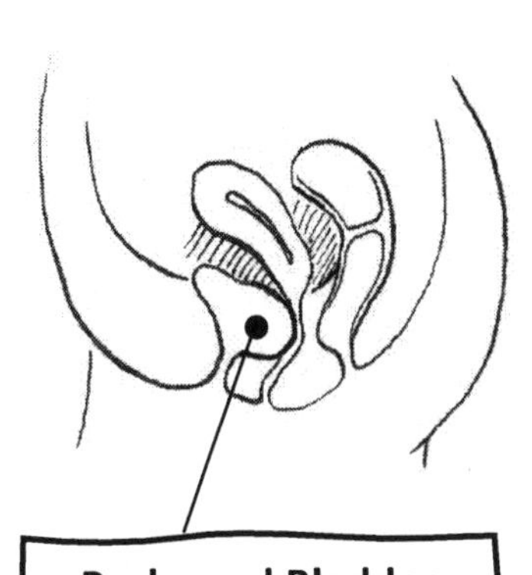

Prolapsed Bladder
also called Cystocele

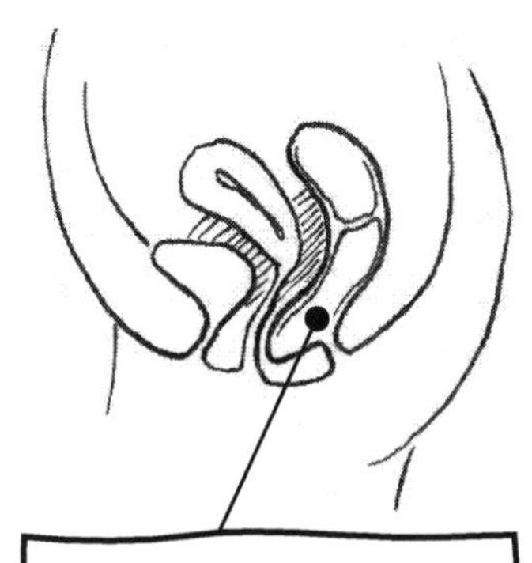

Prolapsed Rectum
also called Rectocele

The process of pelvic organ prolapse may take years, or it can occur immediately after childbirth. Sometimes a new mother arrives in our office, breasts engorged with milk, her baby in a stroller, desperately wanting to understand why her vagina feels the way it does. Other times, a woman may not seek help until her kids leave home, when she is finally able to think about herself again. And some women, even though they have significant prolapse, experience no symptoms at all.

For those fortunate women, surgery is never recommended. Asymptomatic prolapse is not dangerous to your health, and surgery does not help you feel better if you already feel fine.

Anatomically speaking, this is the bottom line: the bladder, the rectum, and the uterus lose their support as the result of delivering a baby. The external appearance of a woman's genitalia changes. The vagina loosens, and the pelvic organs drop down more and more with each passing decade. No one wants to sag. Especially down there.

Sexual dysfunction and changes in appearance are only part of the story of pelvic organ prolapse. Other annoyances may rear their ugly head. A woman with pelvic prolapse can experience herniation of the bladder and urethra resulting in leakage of urine.

What is herniation? Basically, a hernia or herniation is what we call it when an organ protrudes through or out of the cavity in which it normally rests. The word "hernia" comes from the Latin word for "rupture." In this book, I will often use "hernia" and "prolapse" to mean the same thing.

Jumping on a Trampoline

I have not been on a trampoline since I was ten, but for some reason, many women complain that jumping on a trampoline was the first time they noticed urine leakage. (Speaking as an adult who has never looked to jump on trampolines, I've found them easy to avoid.)

But women also experience leaking with coughing, sneezing, laughing, exercise - or even during sexual intercourse. Every week, my office phone rings when a woman in this condition finally decides she has had enough!

Herniation of the rectum is nothing to sneeze at, either (pun intended). Herniation of the rectum, also known as a rectocele, is the condition that results in vaginal looseness for a woman and her partner. A prolapsed rectum can get so bad that a woman has to touch her genitalia to get stool out in the bathroom. In fact, eleven per cent of women have issues with incontinence of feces and gas. This is even worse than urine leakage, because of the odor – and grossness, I suppose. Some women learn to limit the times they leave their homes. It is sad and miserable - but thank God, it's fixable!

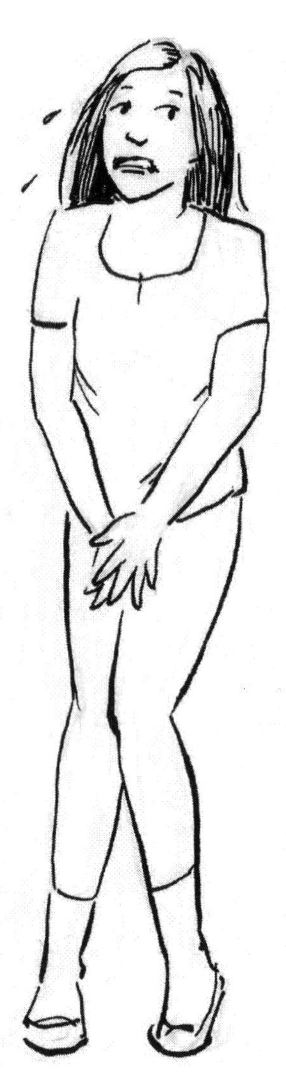

Herniation of the uterus results in pelvic discomfort and pressure that can worsen as the day progresses, or during exercise, or during menstrual cycles. Sex can hurt, too, an ache that occurs during or after sexual intercourse. All this pelvic pain or discomfort contributes to sexual dysfunction.

Who wants to be sexually active if intercourse does not feel good?

A man's interest in sex is not altruistic. I recently saw a patient who needs reconstructive surgery – and a hysterectomy as well. She has severe pain during sex that lasts for days afterward. Yet even though this has been going on for over five years, it has never occurred to her to deny her husband the pleasure of sexual intercourse. Women are strangely beautiful this way – putting others first.

But it is a little mystifying, too. Surely most men would not have sex if it resulted in physical pain. Could you imagine? "This hurts me a lot, honey, but I am doing it for you."

But I Haven't Had a Baby! Why Does My Vagina Feel Loose?

Vaginal looseness, or vaginal laxity, affects many women. It is most common after childbirth, but even women who haven't had children can suffer from it.

Vaginal walls, like the rest of a woman's skin, are made up of collagen and fibrous material that give the skin its strength and flexibility. When a woman goes through a vaginal delivery, she can be overstretched, diminishing both her tightness and sensitivity.

But childbirth isn't the only cause of vaginal laxity. Other causes are:

- Advancing age, which causes the muscles of the body to become more relaxed overall.

- Menopause. About 50% of women report experiencing significant vaginal laxity after menopause because of estrogen levels dropping.

- Trauma to the vagina. Commonly caused by sexual activity with a larger partner, use of large sex toys, or even a history of sexual abuse.

- Genetic disorders that involve collagen metabolism.

For many women who suffer from vaginal laxity, doctors recommend Kegel exercises, which can be done anywhere and are successful in toning the pelvic floor. However, Kegel exercises do nothing to restore the damaged anatomy and connective tissue. These are repaired with pelvic reconstructive surgery.

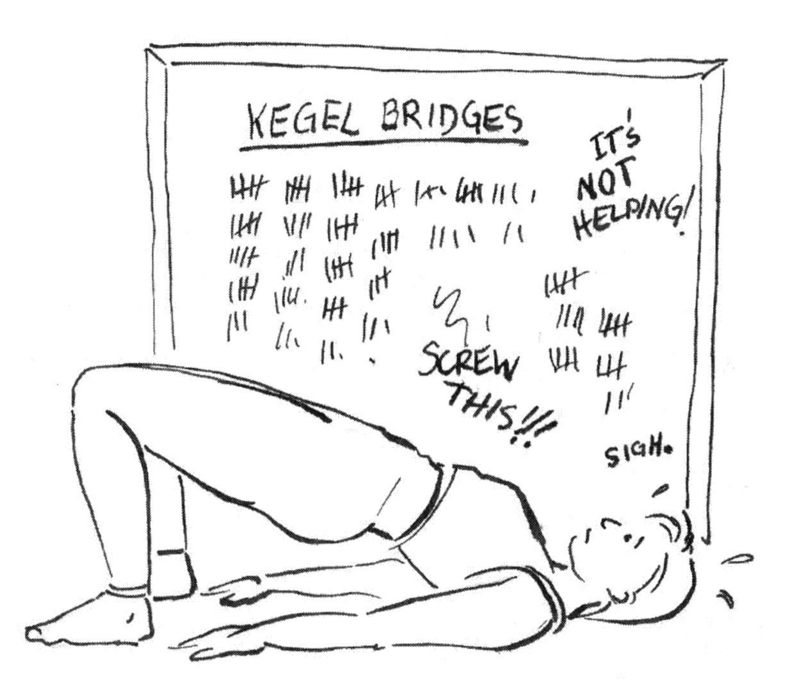
KEGEL BRIDGES
IT'S NOT HELPING!
SCREW THIS!!!
SIGH.

Mirror, Mirror – How To Look

It is important to look at your own anatomy so you can better understand what the outside looks like and get an idea of what is going on inside.

When I do an exam, I ask my patient to hold a hand mirror so she can see her own her anatomy. The labia majora, labia minora, clitoral hood, clitoris, urethra, and vaginal opening are all easy to see.

You can look at home by yourself just as easily.

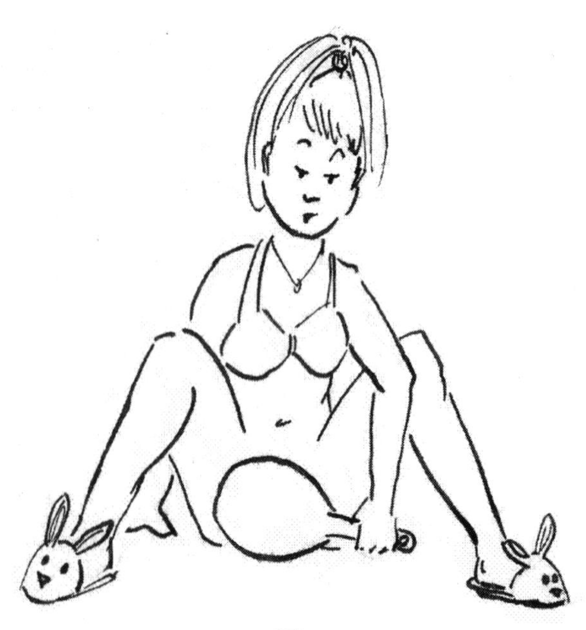

How To Feel What's Going On Inside

You can do this without a mirror. An index finger in your vagina lets you feel the front (anterior) part. The bladder is what you feel with the pad of your finger on the other side of your vaginal wall.

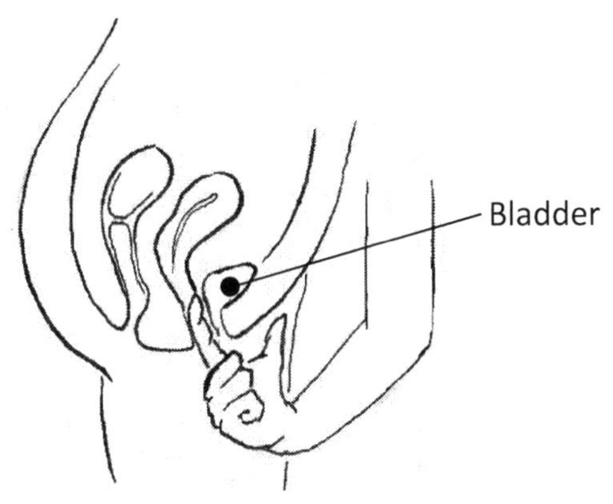

A thumb in your vagina lets you feel the back (posterior) part. The rectum is what you feel with the pad of your thumb through the back vaginal wall.

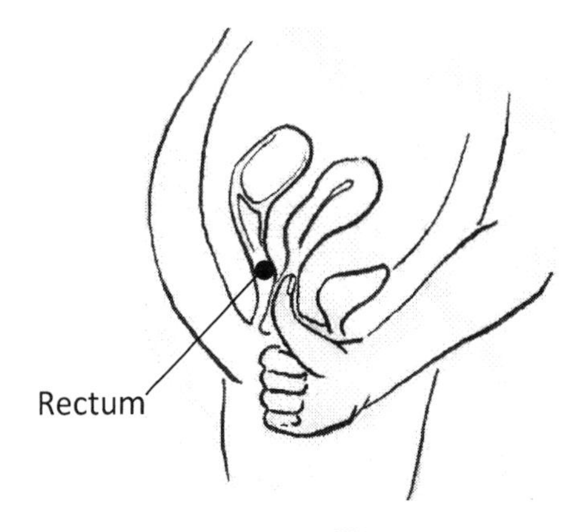

The "Jump Test"

When you cough or bear down, you can also see any organs that are prolapsing. You may feel pressure from your vagina dropping.

Pressure on your index finder means it's the bladder.

Pressure on your thumb, it's the rectum.

If you feel something hitting the tip of your index finger, it's your uterus and/or intestine.

Sexual Feeling – What else can get in the way?

Vaginal laxity and pelvic prolapse aren't the only things that can interfere with your sexual relationship.

Enlarged or distorted labia can interfere with sex, too. In addition, large or drooping labia can also be painful in everyday activities, getting caught in clothing, or preventing you from wearing certain close-fitting styles.

When a woman is self-conscious about her labia, they can even prevent her from having or starting relationships.

Abnormal Labia

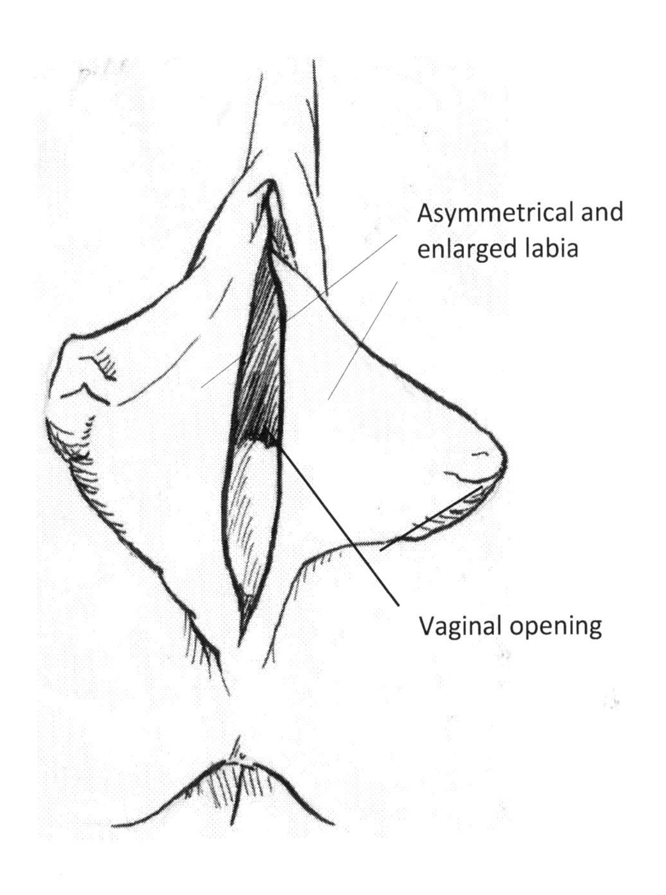

PART 3

Take Control

Understanding How Surgery Can Improve Sex, Your Body, and Your Life

In this section you will learn:

- What you should know about surgery –
and the 3 things the surgeon considers

- GYN problems you should have fixed while you are having cosmetic and reconstructive GYN surgery

- The 4 things that make a vagina tight

- Surgeon's notes – the 3 parts of vaginal tightening

- The basic surgical procedures and how they work
    - Vaginoplasty
    - Labiaplasty of labia minora
    - Labiaplasty of labia majora
    - Clitoral hood reduction
    - Hymenoplasty

- Bladder repair, problems of the uterus, rectal repair

- How to choose a cosmetic GYN surgeon
    - The best type of surgeon for vaginoplasty
    - The best type of surgeon for labiaplasty

Understanding How Surgery Can Improve Sex, Your Body, and Your Life

Surgery can fix some things about your body that nothing else will. However, all surgery has risks. There are two basic things to understand about surgery.

One is, avoid surgery when you can.

Why have your body cut on if you do not have to? It hurts, has risks, and costs money. You sign permission forms that spell out the dangers in fine print, but the bottom line is that going to the operating room is like driving your car on the Interstate. You are trying to get from point A to point B, and you might run into a traffic jam or get into an accident. Be careful!

Two, if surgery is required, only do what is needed, in the safest way possible. Sometimes it means less surgery than you were planning, and sometimes it means more.

These are the three things I want to understand:

1. What do you want to accomplish? Tightness, improved appearance, both?

2. Based on your anatomy, do you actually need surgery, or will an office-based procedure or medication work for you?

3. What other health issues are going on? Have you had painful periods since you were a teen? Do you pass blood clots with your cycles? Does your bladder leak?

Having pelvic surgery is kind of like renovating your house. You might be tired of your kitchen and want an update. Maybe it's just the color of your foyer you hate. Or maybe, the whole foundation of your home is sinking and it's time for a major overhaul.

If there are several problems, it may make sense to fix them all at the same time – as part of your "re-model."

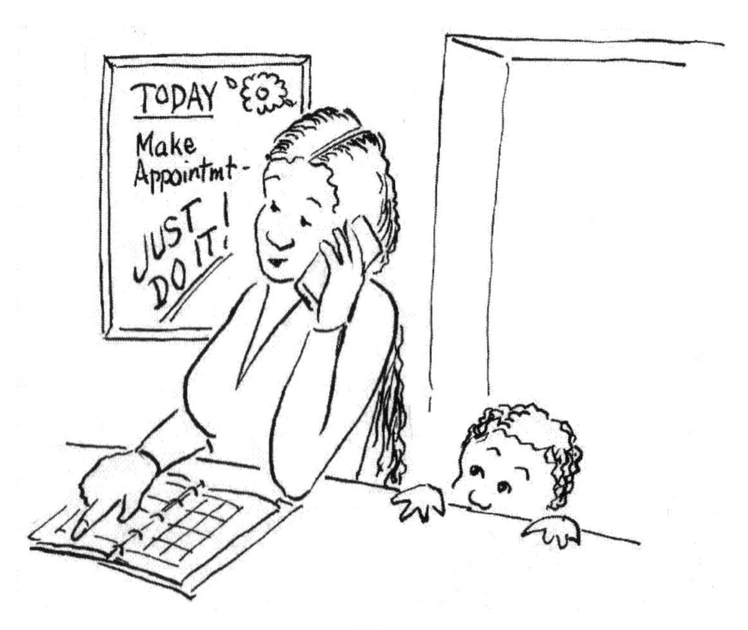

Other GYN Problems To Fix At the Same Time

All surgery is about fixing anatomical problems. The focus of this book is on cosmetic and reconstructive gynecological surgery. Yet many patients seeking this type of surgery have other problems, too, such as bleeding, pelvic pain or bladder leakage.

Surgeons qualified to perform reconstructive GYN surgery (who operate inside the pelvis) can usually address the full range of pelvic and GYN problems. So if you do decide to have surgery, I advise you to have everything taken care of at once. You don't have to suffer.

In this section of the book, I'll talk first about each part of the anatomy, and explain the surgery that can repair damage or correct problems with that part of the body.

Then I will touch briefly on the range of other GYN problems I recommend you address when you are considering cosmetic and reconstructive GYN surgery.

Finally, we will talk about how to choose the best surgeon for your needs.

The Vagina –
4 Things That Make It Tight

The vagina is the fibromuscular tube leading to the uterus or womb. It is the receptacle for the penis during sexual intercourse, where semen is deposited at ejaculation to allow for pregnancy and the passageway for the newborn.

Looseness of the vagina means there is less friction during sexual intercourse. This diminishes sensation for both partners.

So what does it mean to be "tight"? There are 4 components of vaginal tightness:

1. The size of your opening and your vaginal canal.
2. The strength of your pelvic floor muscles.
3. The amount of lubrication you secrete.
4. The size of your partner.

Surgery addresses only the first one – the size of the opening and the vaginal canal. Repair of the opening is called a perineoplasty. Repair of the vaginal canal is called a vaginoplasty. But they should always be done at the same time. Why have a tight opening and loose canal, or vice versa?

The Vaginal Opening

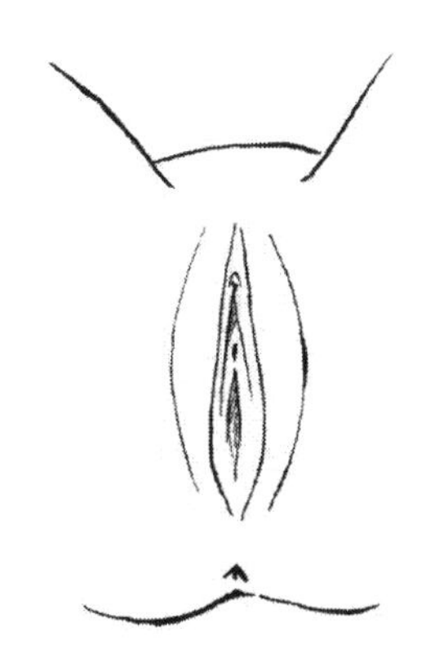

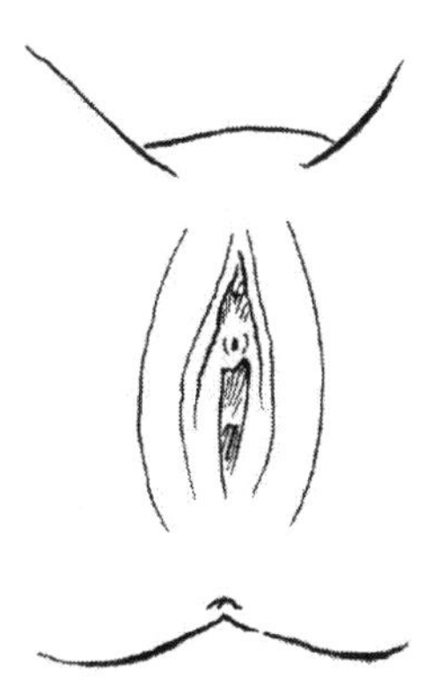

Before Sex - Virginal

After Sexual Relations

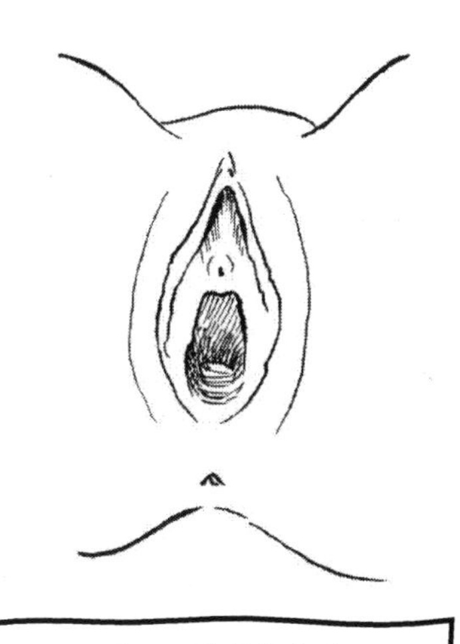

After Childbirth

The Vaginal Canal

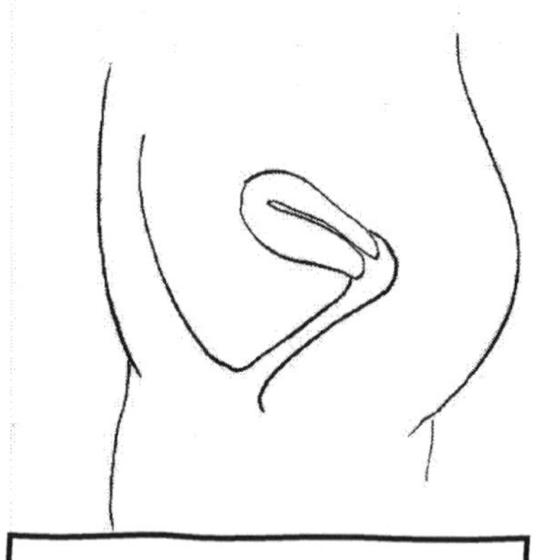

Before Sex – Virginal
(one to two fingers' width)

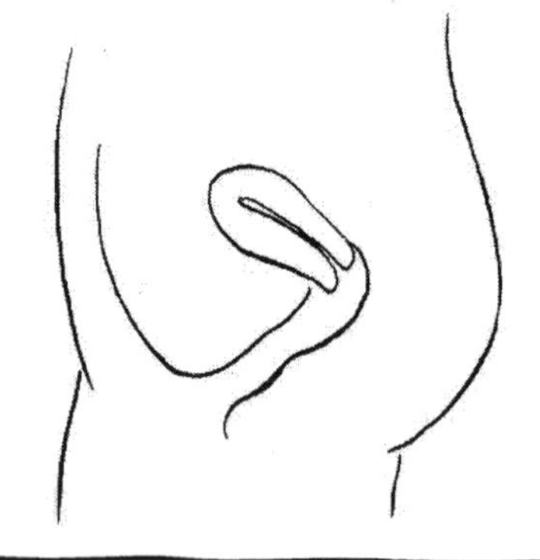

After Sexual Relations
(two to three fingers' width)

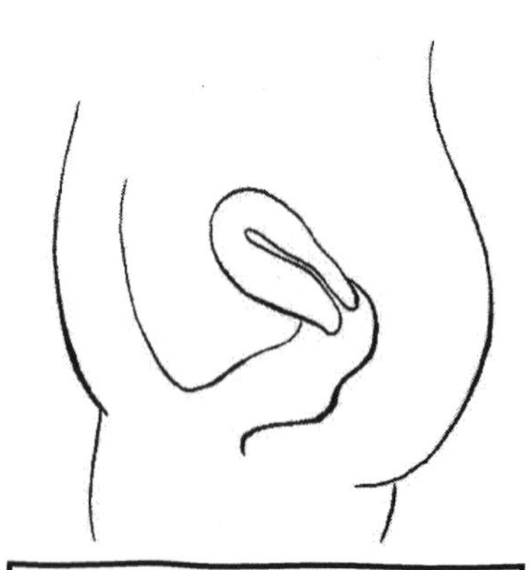

After Childbirth
(three to five fingers' width)

Surgical Tightening for the Loose Vagina – What Do You Call It?

The medical words used to describe cosmetic GYN and reconstructive pelvic surgery can be confusing. Since it's a new surgical subspecialty, there are not established definitions, or even a precise, formal training process (yet).

The most confusing term of all is "Vaginal Rejuvenation." Vaginal Rejuvenation is an unfortunate marketing term coined twenty years ago, and is not even correct medical terminology.

When words are not clear, communication is poor.

This is what women want to know: Will just the opening to the vagina be tightened, or will it be the entire canal?

Because there is so much confusion about vaginal tightening, even among surgeons who sometimes perform this procedure, I'll describe my surgical technique for vaginal tightening. I will use the medical terms for the three component parts of the procedure. If this section is more technical than you want, feel free to skip directly to page 99, "More About Tightness."

(And YES! The tightening is for the whole canal.)

Surgeon's Notes

The Three Parts of Vaginal Tightening

There are three components to tightening your vagina:

1. **Perineoplasty** – tightening the vaginal opening

2. **Rectocele repair** (also known as **posterior colporrhaphy**) – fixing the prolapsed rectum behind the vagina

3. **Vaginoplasty** – tightening the vaginal canal

First the Perineoplasty

Vaginal tightening begins with addressing the vaginal opening. This part of the surgery is known as a perineoplasty. A physical exam helps determine the original condition of your anatomy before you had children or became sexually active. (How much tighter were you? What was the original size of your vaginal opening?) The tissue on the outside is marked to determine the future, smaller size of your opening.

An incision is made, and the musculature of your opening is exposed. Any unattractive or damaged skin on the outside is removed.

The perineoplasty exposes your perineal body, the central tendon positioned between the opening of your vagina and your anus. This is where the muscles of your openings meet. The names of these muscles include the ischiocavernosus and bulbospongiosus muscles, the transverse perineal muscles, the anal sphincter, the posterior vaginal muscularis, and the levator ani muscles.

These are shown in the illustration on the next page. *(Notes continued on p. 100)*

External Muscles for

Perineoplasty

(surgery for vaginal opening)

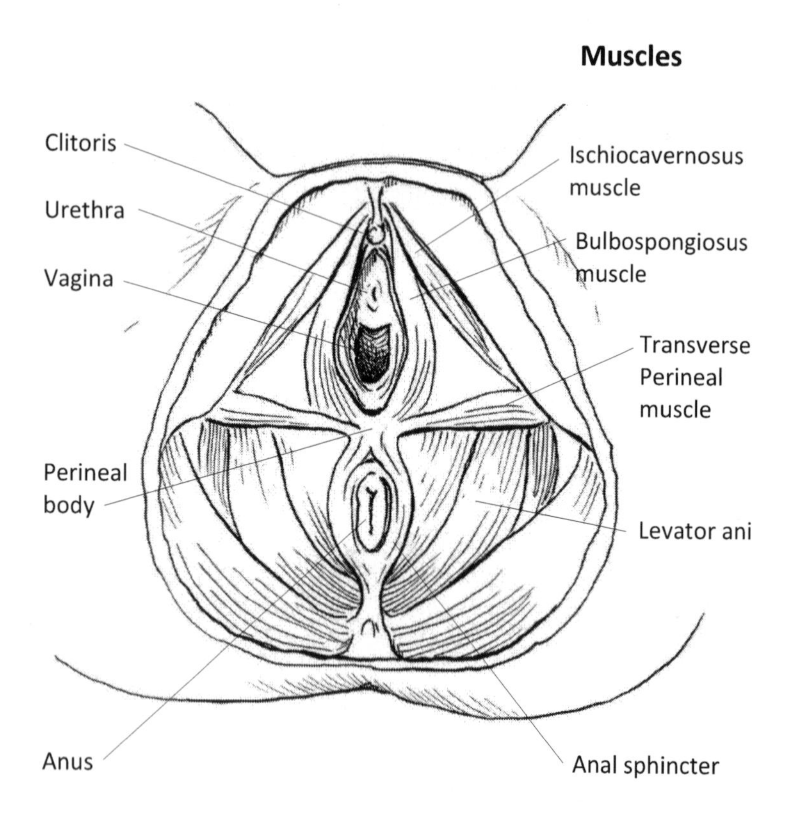

Deeper Muscles for

Vaginoplasty

(surgery for vaginal canal)

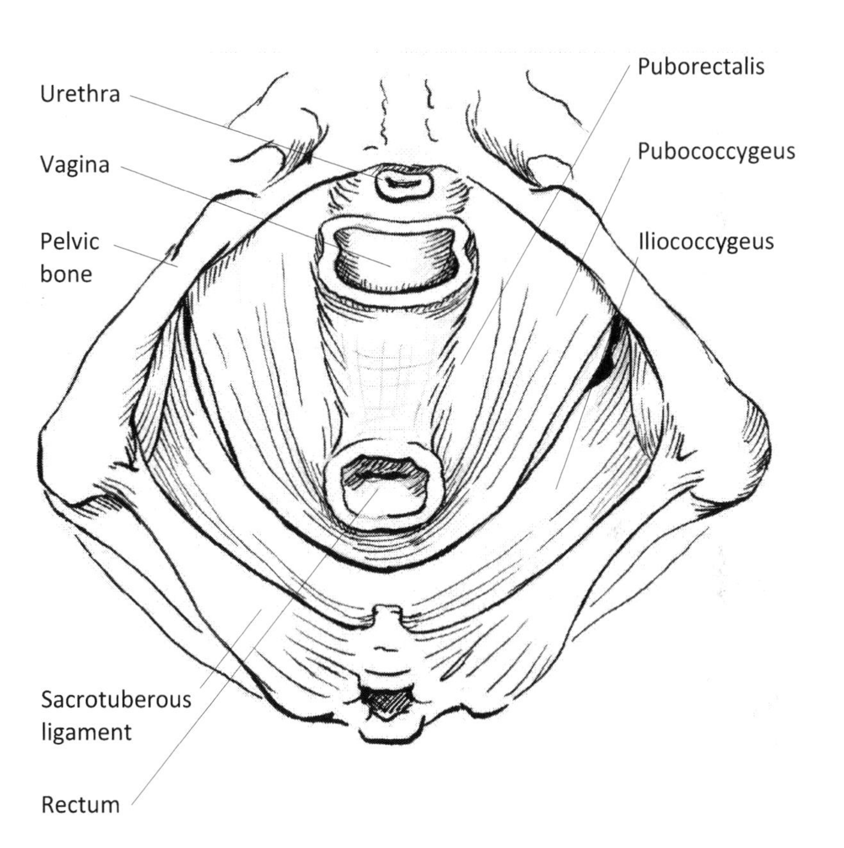

Surgeon's Notes, cont.

The Three Parts of Vaginal Tightening

Repair the Prolapsed Rectum (Rectocele)

Once the perineoplasty is begun, your anatomy is exposed and visible. It's time to start the vaginoplasty to tighten the canal.

You might be interested to know that tightness in your vaginal opening and canal comes from the posterior (back) part of your pelvis – the part you would feel with your thumb.

The back side of the vagina is typically opened in the midline and separated from the underlying rectum. There is always a prolapse here in the rectum (a rectocele) that must be repaired before the vagina is tightened. The rectum is protruding through the vagina, which is why a rectocele is also known as a "herniated" rectum. The protrusion is the bulge you can feel when you insert your thumb in your vagina.

The rectocele is almost always a transverse (side-to-side) break of the underlying fibromuscular vaginal tissue. It's not the skin of the vagina that is damaged, but the fibromuscular foundation, called the rectovaginal fascia.

You can actually see the break if you look closely at your vaginal canal with a mirror! Where the back side of the vagina is wrinkled, it means there is intact fascia underneath the vaginal skin. Where the vagina is smooth, there is no fascia present, only rectum underneath. This is where the break is.

Once the fascia is identified, it is sutured to where it originally was positioned at the top and the sides. From a surgical perspective, this means reattaching the fascia to the back of the cervix, where there are ligaments that attach the uterus to the hollow of your pelvis or sacrum. This also means reattaching the fascia laterally to the side wall musculature. (The sutures dissolve on their own after about six weeks and do not have to be removed.)

This completes the repair of the rectocele.

(The step I describe above - reattaching the fascia - is often neglected by reconstructive GYN surgeons. Pelvic herniations involve several organ systems in a three dimensional space, and reattaching broken fascia requires deep dissection into the body. It can be technically challenging. Even now, after completing thousands of pelvic reconstruction cases, I still routinely seek to refine my technique to perfect the surgery.)

Completing the Vaginoplasty

In the final step of vaginal tightening, the vaginoplasty portion is completed. The good news is that the vagina at this point is again intact. The bad news is that the tissue around it (the rectovaginal fascia) is often badly stretched and weakened, broken by childbirth (and sex). The levator ani muscles, which give tightness to the vagina, are inevitably damaged as well. Painstaking layers of suture are done in this stage of the surgery to repair the damaged fascia and muscles, re-establishing the tightness of the vaginal tube.

With the vaginal canal narrowed, excess vaginal skin is removed and the vagina is closed with suture all the way out to the opening. The muscles of the perineal body are sutured back together. The skin on the outside is then closed, finished with fine suture for the best appearance.

And More About Tightness...

How far does the tightness extend?

The tightness always extends at least two thirds of the way up your vaginal canal. The top third of your vagina is naturally hollow because it acts as reservoir to hold semen after ejaculation. There is no adjacent musculature at the top one third that can be repaired. Some women show more hollowness at the top of their vagina than others. The top one third is tightened back to the way it was. But since there is no surrounding muscle – depending on the structure of your anatomy - it may not be as tight as the lower two thirds of your vagina.

How tight do you become?

Most of my patients want to be as tight as they were before they were sexually active. This makes sense because once the patient resumes sexual activity after healing from surgery, she will become looser, just as she did when she was first sexually active. However, she will not become as loose as she did from having children and/or the aging process.

The degree of tightness is determined by the shape of her pelvis. A vaginoplasty will restore a woman's body back to the way it was during teenage years but will not create additional tightness. Some women are tighter than others, just like men are different sizes.

In general, a woman who seeks out surgery to tighten her vagina can accommodate four fingers inserted into her vagina during an exam. After the surgery, her vagina is tightened so that it accommodates about a finger and a half.

What do you do if you are not tight enough?

This is not a common complaint, but one I always have attention on. Tightness comes in large part from repairing the anatomy. But sometimes the muscles must also be strengthened. You can think about it this way: If you break the bone of your arm and require surgery, the bone will eventually heal. But will your arm be as strong? Probably not. The muscles will have to be built back.

For pelvic musculature, there are the classic Kegel exercises and pelvic floor physical therapy. It is rare to require a repeat vaginoplasty in the absence of activity that damages your vagina (such as having another child or a large partner or the use of large sex toys).

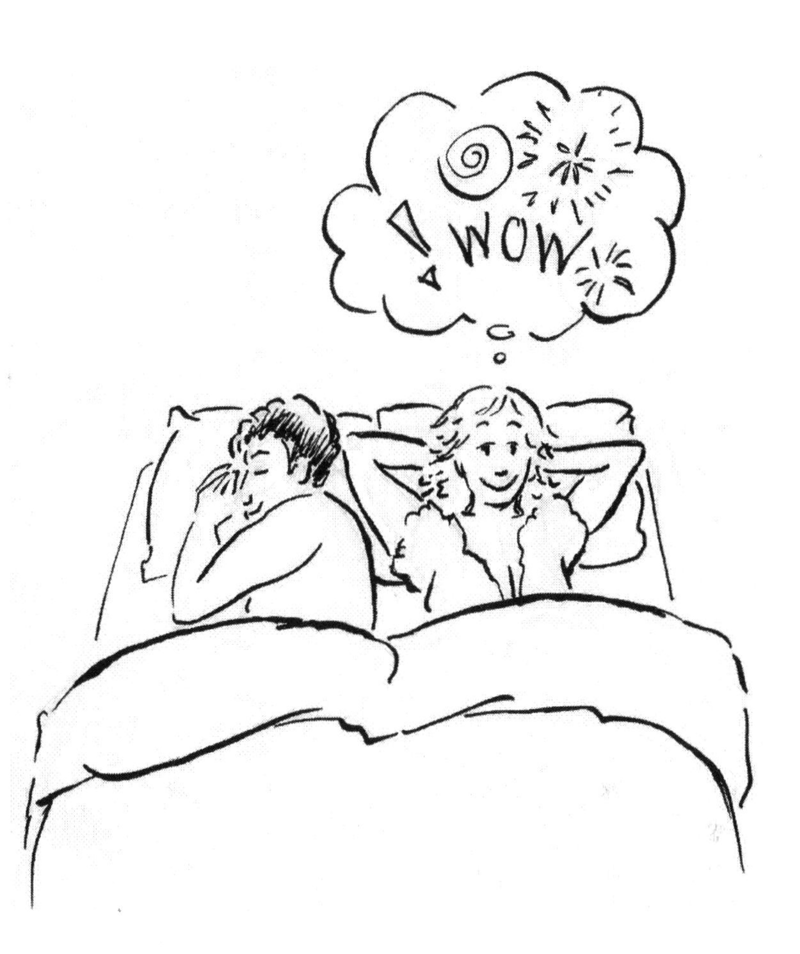
WOW

Labia Minora

The labia minora or "small lips" are two flaps of skin on either side of the opening to the vagina, just inside the labia majora (or large lips). They extend from the clitoris down toward your perineal body.

Labiaplasty – Surgical Repair of Enlarged Labia Minora

The common complaint about the labia minora is that the lips are too large and hang out too far. This can cause discomfort with clothing or with sex, or appear as an undesired esthetic feature.

Typically, a woman will consider her labia enlarged if they extend over the outer lips (labia majora). Some women do not like the dark pigmentation that may become more prominent with pregnancy and aging.

Surgical repair of the labia is called a labiaplasty. The procedure is well tolerated by most women. There is typically no loss of sensation.

I don't recommend that the labia minora be removed entirely, as is done in the "barbie look." The usual practice is to reduce them in size so the edges just meet the labia majora. This gives a balanced esthetic appearance.

Of course, esthetic goals should be tailored to a woman's desire. But it is important to blend the labia minora from the hood of the clitoris downward. In other words, depending on the shape of your anatomy, extra skin left at the top ensures that the structure of your clitoris does not become prominent (like a little penis).

Labiaplasty

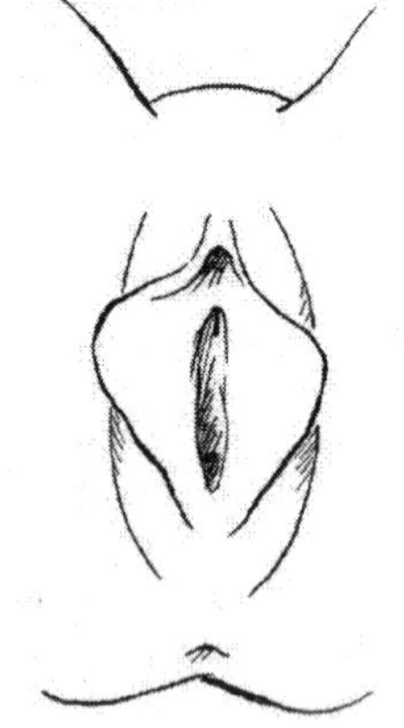

Labia Minora Before Surgery

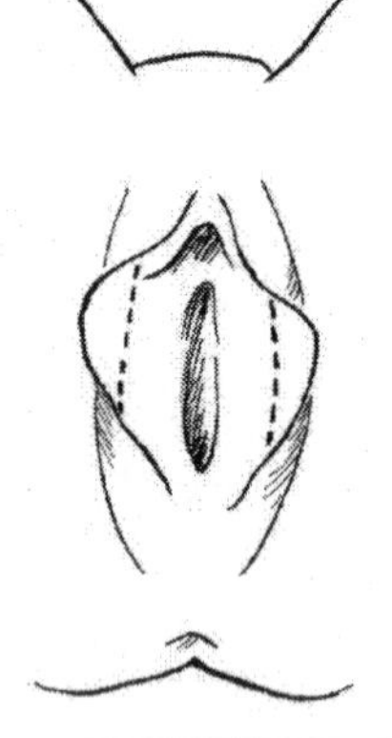

Labia Minora with Surgical Markings
(tissue to be removed)

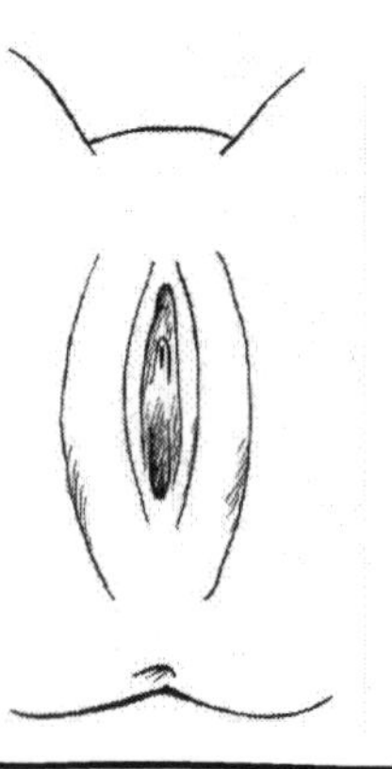

Labia Minora After Surgery

The Labia Majora

The labia majora, or "large lips," are the prominent skin folds on the outside of either side of your vaginal opening. The labia majora extend from your mons down to your perineal body, the area between your vaginal opening and your anus.

Majoraplasty – Surgical Repair of Labia Majora

The typical problem women have with their labia majora is dissatisfaction with their appearance. The labia majora become saggy and wrinkled with childbirth and aging. The skin is no longer tight and can easily be stretched up to two inches or more. This condition is related to decreased structural proteins and loss of fat volume with aging, as well as with childbirth damage.

Surgical repair of this area is straightforward. The operation is called a labiaplasty of the labia majora, or majoraplasty. Excess skin is removed from either side – like a tummy tuck of the labia majora – and the underlying tissue is reconstructed. The incision should be strategically placed so the scar blends in naturally and is not noticed. Women find the procedure tolerable for the simple reason that the labia majora are biologically designed to be stretched and abused during the birth of a baby. The labia majora are a resilient and powerful tissue.

Fat Transfer Into the Labia Majora

Some women with labia majora deflated from loss of fat may benefit from a fat transfer from another part of their body, such as the inner thighs, flank or abdomen. If liposuction of those areas is not planned, other fillers can be used. A hyaluronic acid product such as Juvederm, or platelet rich plasma (PRP) isolated from a simple blood draw, are examples of other fillers commonly used.

Majoraplasty

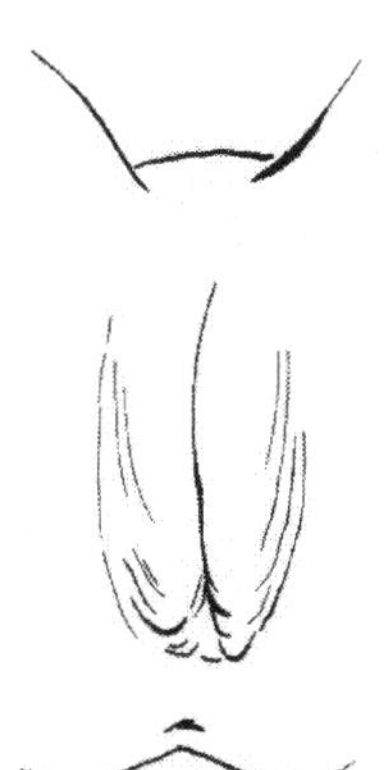

Labia Majora
Before Surgery

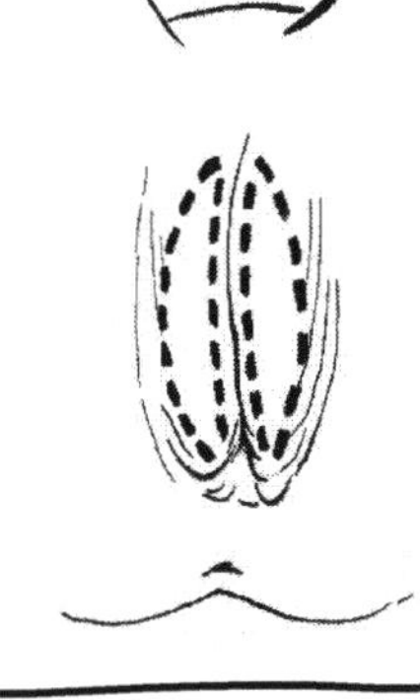

Labia Majora
with Surgical Markings
(tissue to be removed)

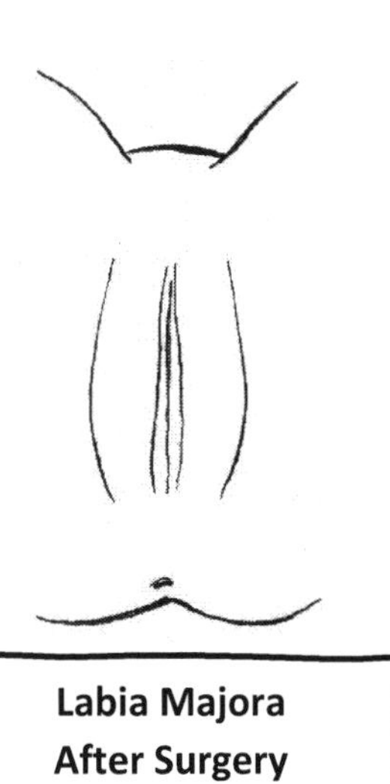

Labia Majora
After Surgery

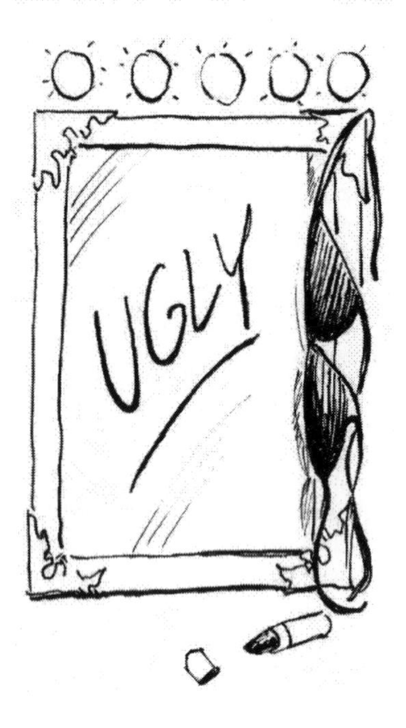

Patient Story

Humiliated by My Body

"I was in high school. I thought I looked great in my new black bikini. There was a guy there I had a crush on. I wanted to impress him. My nails were done and I had nice sunglasses and my hair back. And some jerk pointed at my crotch and told everyone it looked like I had "a little penis." Everybody laughed.

I ran home and I cried for hours. I never knew there was anything wrong with me. But I never felt good about the way I looked again. I never wore a bathing suit again or went to parties. I figured everyone was laughing at me and talking about me. I could hardly look in the mirror.

A few years ago, Dr. Litrel fixed my body. I was engaged to be married and was worried my fiancé would be disgusted by me on our wedding night. But the labiaplasty changed my life. I no longer felt shame. I felt beautiful again like I used to feel.

Now that we have children and all that worry is behind me, I think maybe that experience served a purpose. I didn't sleep around during high school or college like most girls did. I would have, but I was too ashamed of myself.

My husband really is glad that I saved myself for him. I am, too. It's funny how things work out."

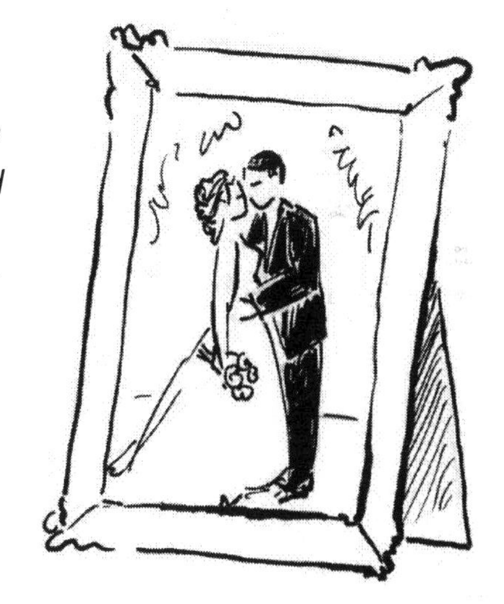

The Clitoral Hood

The clitoral hood, also known as the clitoral prepuce, is the fold of skin that covers the external shaft of the clitoris and a portion of the glans (the head of the clitoris). In some women, the glans of the clitoris is completely covered. This can result in sexual dysfunction.

Surgical Repair – A Clitoral Hood Reduction

The most common procedure performed on the clitoral hood is a reduction. In this situation, there is extra skin that is typically lateral to (on either side of) the clitoral hood, emanating from the labia minora below. You can see the anatomy with a hand mirror at home, or take a look during your office visit.

The extra skin in the clitoral hood is removed at the time of labiaplasty of the minora. Surgical removal of excess skin is performed so that about 3 millimeters of the glans of the clitoris is showing. Oftentimes with this procedure, sagging skin of the prepuce is repaired at the same time.

Clitoral hood reduction is easy to understand when you see in a hand mirror the excess skin outlined by a marker.

Extension of the Clitoral Hood

This procedure can be required when too much of the clitoris shows. This is common with women who get testosterone pellets. Rare ovarian or adrenal gland tumors may also cause this issue. Ideally, 3 millimeters of the glans shows in a non-aroused state. However, testosterone enlarges the glans, and the larger it becomes, the more it resembles a small penis. These changes do not recede once the testosterone pellets are stopped.

With surgery, the skin of the prepuce can be extended to cover an enlarged clitoral glans.

Clitoral Hood Reduction

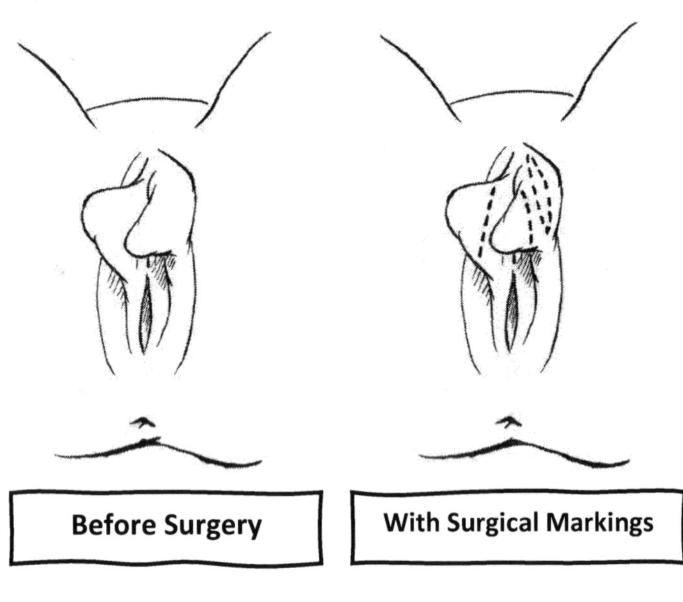

Before Surgery

With Surgical Markings

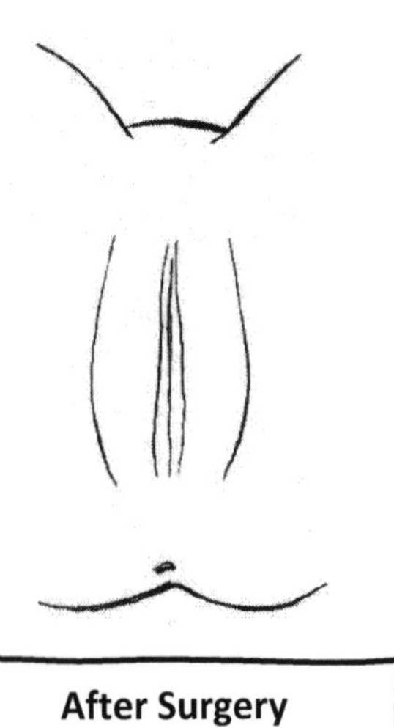

After Surgery

The Hymen

The hymen is a thin membrane of skin that surrounds or partially covers the opening of the vagina. It is the part that is "broken" during the "loss of virginity" – or sometimes with the use of sex toys or tampons.

Surgical Repair of the Hymen

The classic medical condition requiring surgery on the hymen are those cases involving young women with overdeveloped hymens who are unable to pass the blood from their vagina during menstruation. This is called an imperforate hymen – or a hymen without a perforation. Menstrual blood builds up in the vagina because it cannot exit. This is easily addressed surgically. It is not that common.

Restoring Virginity - the Hymenoplasty

The more common reason for hymen surgery today is restoration of virginity. This procedure is called a hymenoplasty. Women who seek this surgery typically belong to a culture that demands virginity at the time of marriage. Women in these cultures are expected to bleed on their wedding day.

This is always a sensitive issue. Women who seek this surgery are often frightened and desperate. There must be blood on the bedsheets on the day of the wedding.

I personally do not condone cultural standards that control women in an authoritarian or suppressive manner. However, I am sensitive to the fact that women in this situation sometimes find themselves trapped by the expectations of family and their community. When they agree to marry, their past sexual history can make a hymenoplasty a desired surgical intervention.

A critical feature of the surgery is that any scars cannot be noticed. Many woman are evaluated before their wedding day by family members of the groom, or even doctors, and are certainly evaluated by the groom after the wedding.

Usually the women on whom I have performed hymenoplasties grew up in America or Europe where the sexual mores are less stringent, but are marrying into their parents' more traditional ethnic culture.

A woman who falls into this category must understand that restoring her anatomical virginity is the only thing accomplished by surgery. I can repair her body so it bleeds on the wedding night. But she, of course, will need to supply any virginal role playing on the wedding night. In these scenarios, the occasion is often a tense and frightening experience for the bride.

Again, I do not believe women should be placed under this pressure. I am just aware that many are – and I am able to help.

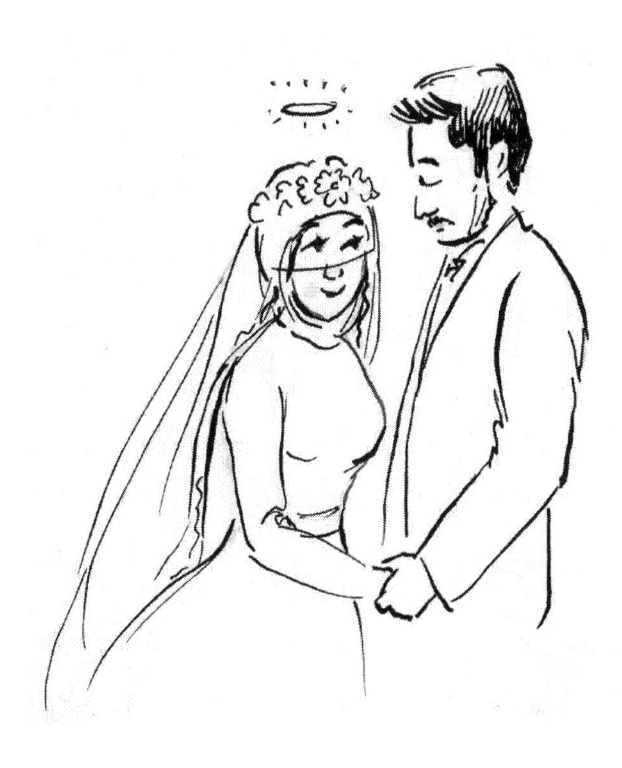

Will I bleed on my wedding day?

This is the key question for every patient seeking this surgery.

Traditionally, surgeons tell women that bleeding is not guaranteed after hymenoplasty. This is true in the sense that not all women bleed the first time they are sexually active. Some hymens are thin and open and don't have good blood supply. These are the hymens that won't bleed. When a hymen is restored surgically, there is even less blood supply because of the scarring associated with healing from surgical repair. This is why women are warned they may not bleed.

But if bleeding on the wedding day is the point of having the surgery, why have the surgery if it's not guaranteed?

I have modified the surgery for those seeking a hymenoplasty so that bleeding will certainly occur. Yes, nothing is guaranteed in life – but I have not had any failures to date. I have also not had any repaired hymens break during the healing process before the wedding day. Any surgical wound can break apart. The tissue of the hymen is so thin that physical activity during the healing process can result in bleeding before the wedding day, not on the day.

How Is bleeding guaranteed?

The key to surgical success with a "wedding-night hymenoplasty" is to tighten the vaginal canal above the hymen. Tightening of the vaginal opening itself is avoided to prevent any scars which might show on the wedding day, or in a medical evaluation scheduled beforehand to confirm virginity.

Once the vaginal canal above the hymen is reconstructed and tightened, the hymen is then surgically restored. Since the hymen rests just outside the tightened vaginal canal, it will heal without breaking before the wedding day. The thin tissue of the hymen is resting on a basement of the strong, tight vaginal canal.

On the wedding day, the hymen and vagina will be so tight that even the smallest penis can't enter without blood on the bedsheets.

The Mons Pubis

The mons pubis, also known as the mons or pubic mound, is a rounded mass of fatty tissue covering the pubic bone at the top of the external genitalia. It has hair, and is the part of your genitalia you see when you are standing in front of the mirror.

Monsplasty – Surgical Repair of the Mons

Some women have troublesome sagging of their mons. A mons lift can be performed to remove excess skin and fat and to give a more esthetic appearance.

Excess fat on the mons often extends to the labia majora. In this case, liposuction of the mons can be performed independently, or at the same time as a mons lift.

Liposuction of the mons is sometimes performed at the time of a tummy tuck or abdominoplasty. Care must be taken when combining these procedures, because there can be distortion of the labia majora if they are not done correctly.

Less common issues with the mons occur with excess lifting during abdominoplasty, distorting the anatomy. Correction requires release of the skin and reconstruction of the tummy tuck incision. Sometimes a fat transfer into the mons is required as well.

Monsplasty

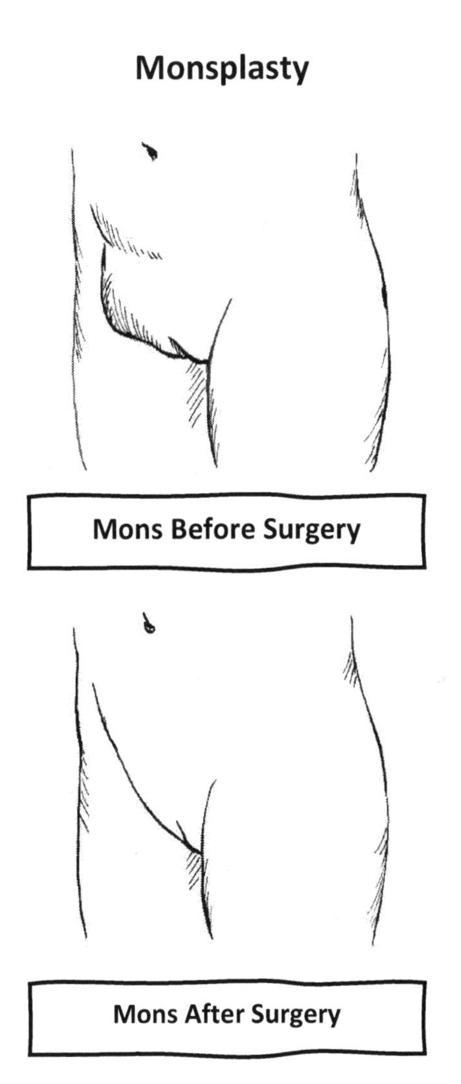

The Female Orgasm System and Surgery

The erogenous areas of a woman's body responsible for the female orgasm are the clitoris and the G-spot. Typically, these areas are not damaged by childbirth because they are protected by the pubic bone.

However, nerves can become less sensitive as we age. For example, when you were a child, putting asparagus or pepper in your mouth may have caused you distress. Your taste buds were too sensitive. But as you got older, you might have found you enjoyed these flavors more. Your taste buds became less sensitive, so the flavor stimulation was more pleasurable.

Similarly, the nerves of sexual responsiveness lessen in sensitivity with age. How can you repair those nerves? You assist the body to heal itself! Encouraging regrowth of the clitoral nerves and those of the G-spot can be done with a process that injects growth factors, harvested from your own blood, into the area surrounding your genitals to assist rejuvenation of the nerves.

For this treatment, your own blood is used, the growth factors within it isolated using a centrifuge and specialized test tube. The resulting platelet rich plasma is what is used as an injection. This technique is known as the O shot®.

Location of the G-spot

(anterior vaginal wall)

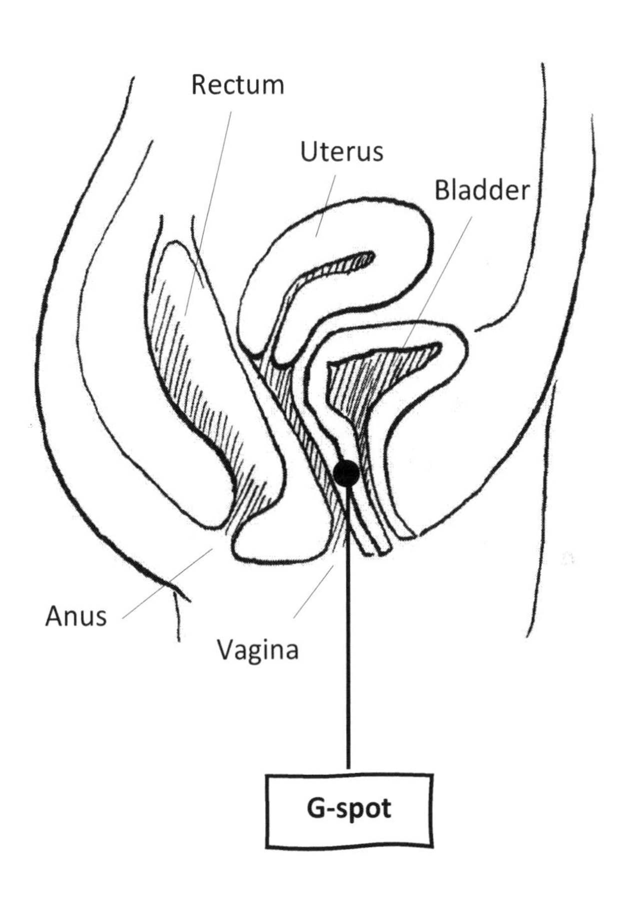

Common Repairs to Have Done When You Have Cosmetic GYN and Reconstructive Surgery

Many women who seek help with cosmetic gynecology have related issues with pelvic health or prolapse. Ideally, these should be addressed during the cosmetic GYN and reconstructive surgery. The issues include: bladder repair, repair of a prolapsed rectum (a rectocele), and problems with the uterus, including prolapse, pain, and bleeding.

The following is a brief overview of those problems with an explanation of their repair.

Bladder Repair

The bladder is the organ that stores your urine. It is a muscle that contracts when you are ready to void (or empty) urine from your body. Common problems include prolapse of the bladder and leakage. Prolapse of the bladder is repaired surgically. This is called an anterior colporrhaphy, or repair of cystocele.

Lifting the Urethra

The urethra is the tube that leads from the bladder to the outside. You can see the opening by spreading your labia minora. It is a small slit located just above your vaginal opening. If you cough or bear down and the urethra moves, you may have what is called a urethrocele (prolapsed urethra). Excessive mobility of the urethra is what causes women to leak urine when they sneeze or engage in physical activity.

With a urethrocele, the issue is simply this: activity causes the bladder to drop and the urethra to move. This means there is increased pressure inside your bladder and decreased pressure keeping your urethra closed. It's this pressure difference that causes the leakage. The urine leaking out of the urethra is comparable to air escaping from a balloon when you let go of the stem.

The bladder leakage can be surgically repaired. A sling made of polypropylene mesh is inserted in such a way to lift up the urethra so it no longer leaks. This type of sling is considered the gold standard treatment for fixing urinary incontinence of this type.

However, there are class action law suits involving a product related to the sling, called transvaginal mesh. Since the companies that make the urethral slings also made the transvaginal mesh, trial attorneys have initiated lawsuits which include everything, including the slings.

For severe incontinence, the midurethral sling produces the best results. However, for patients with mild cases, or for those who worry about slings, I sometimes use an alternative technique for the repair which uses sutures alone.

Bladder Repair

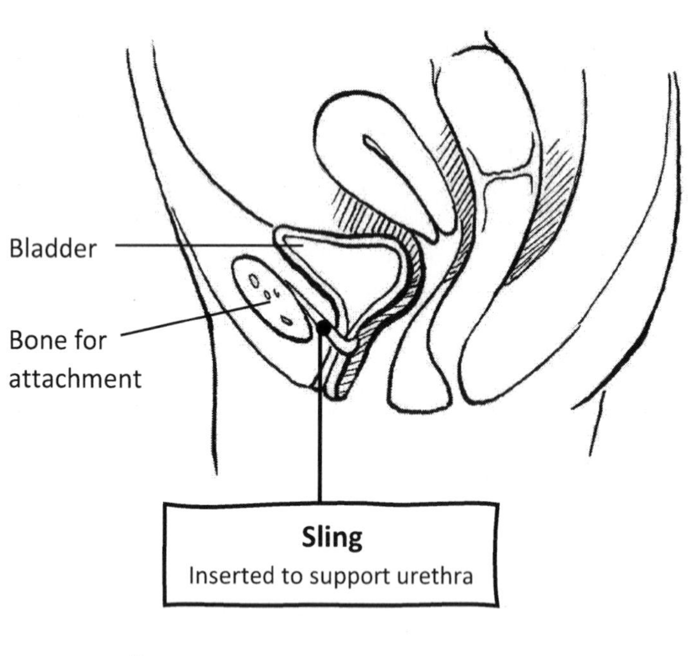

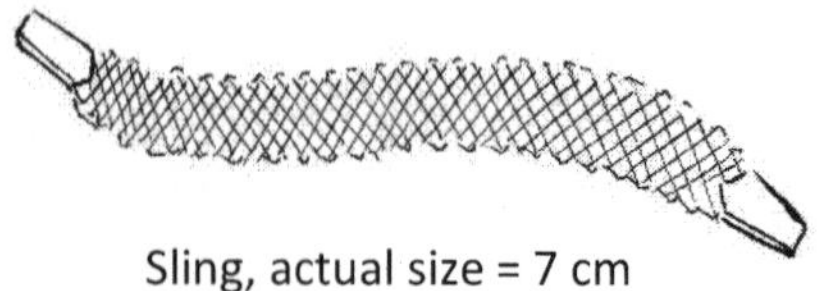

Sling, actual size = 7 cm

Repair of the Rectum

The rectum is where you store your stool before defecation. Prolapse of the rectum is called a rectocele. A rectocele repair, also known as a posterior colporrhaphy, is the surgery required. This is always done (as described earlier) before the performance of a vaginoplasty.

The Cervix

The cervix is the lowest part of the uterus, located at the top of the vagina. It can be seen by the doctor during a medical exam using an instrument called a speculum. The cervix is the part of the uterus that dilates (opens up) when you are in labor.

A common problem of the cervix is with infections such as chlamydia, gonorrhea, and human papilloma virus. These are sexually transmitted infections. The human papilloma virus, or HPV, can cause both genital warts and cervical cancer. The purpose of Pap smears is to make certain you do not have cancer or lesions that may lead to cancer. Before you have any surgery of your genitalia, it is important to make sure any problem of your cervix is correctly diagnosed and treated, including sexually transmitted diseases.

Problems of the Uterus - Prolapse, Pain and Bleeding

The uterus, or womb, is the organ in which your baby grows and the organ that sheds menstrual blood. Common problems with the uterus include bleeding, pain, and prolapse. A long history of menstrual pain or cramping since your teenage years may indicate a common issue called endometriosis. If pain and bleeding started in your adult years, you will need evaluation for fibroids, which are benign muscle tumors of the uterus.

Prolapse of the uterus should be addressed surgically when vaginal tightening procedures are performed. The uterus can be suspended so it stays inside of your body. But if you have significant pain with your cycles or with sex, a hysterectomy or removal of your uterus should be considered.

If your issue is only heavy cycles and you are finished having children, a simple procedure called an endometrial ablation is a good alternative to a hysterectomy. An ablation is a procedure where the lining of the uterus is removed so you no longer have cycles, or your bleeding is greatly reduced.

The bottom line is simply this: when you are considering cosmetic gynecology, make certain all your gynecological issues are addressed.

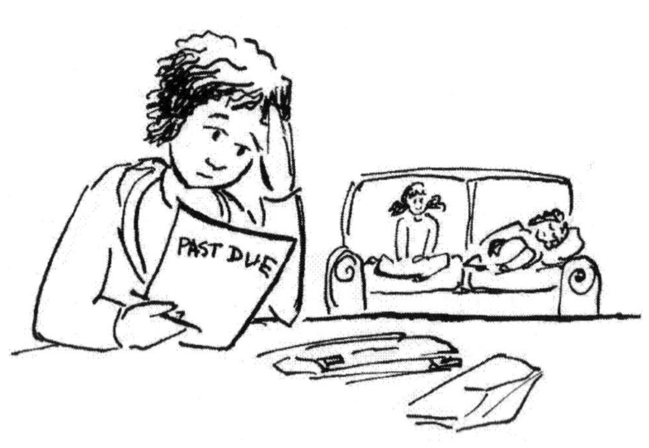

Patient Story

Courage to Start Over Again

"Before the divorce, I worked two jobs while my ex was in school. Then when he finally started making money, he ran off with a younger woman and started a whole new family.

He didn't even care enough to see our daughters. He never paid his child support, even though he could have afforded it. It took me a long time to get over all the anger.

After the girls graduated high school, I had met someone and I was considering a relationship. But I was afraid to take it to the next level.

Having babies did a lot of damage. I leaked. I looked terrible. Everything sagged. I wasn't the woman I used to be.

I got to Dr. Litrel's office, and I hated looking at myself in that mirror.

But he told me it was all normal and all fixable. This was really the first time I felt like I could let myself hope.

After I recovered, my body looked great, and I stopped leaking. I got up the courage to start a relationship. Sex was better than it ever was. It was so much worth the wait! We are talking about getting married."

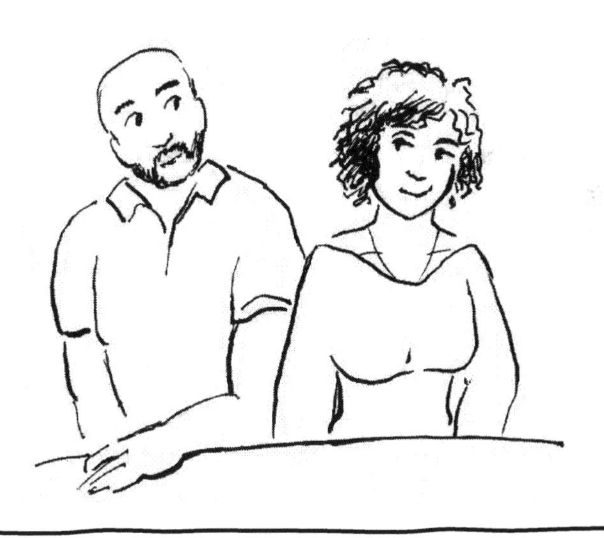

How To Choose Your Surgeon

I prefer you choose me as your surgeon. But sadly, I cannot fix everyone. If you and I never build a doctor patient relationship, this section is about choosing the right surgeon for you.

Obviously, personal rapport, price, and proximity matter. You want to feel good about your surgeon, not pay out your nose, and not travel too far. Right? But above all, you want to choose a skilled surgeon. When it comes to surgery, do it right the first time – or don't do it at all.

The key to choosing a skilled surgeon is to find out about their experience and training. But this can be confusing. What exactly is a surgeon – is that the same as a medical doctor, or a specialist? How does he or she get experience and training?

All doctors go to medical school and study four years of basic medical science to earn their Doctorate in Medicine, the MD degree. Afterward, a doctor will train for many more years to specialize in their area of interest. In the case of surgeons, this can mean an additional four to eight years of training after graduation from medical school.

There are three types of surgeons who perform cosmetic gynecological surgery:

General Obstetricians and Gynecologists (FACOG)
Urogynecologist (FPMRS)
Plastic surgeons (FACS)

All these doctors have "MD" after their name, meaning "Medical Doctor." FACOG stands for "Fellow of American College of Obstetrics and Gynecology." This is your OB-GYN. FPMRS stands for "Fellow of Female Pelvic Medicine and Reconstructive Surgery." This is your Urogynecologist. And FACS is "Fellow of the American College of Surgeons." This is your plastic surgeon.

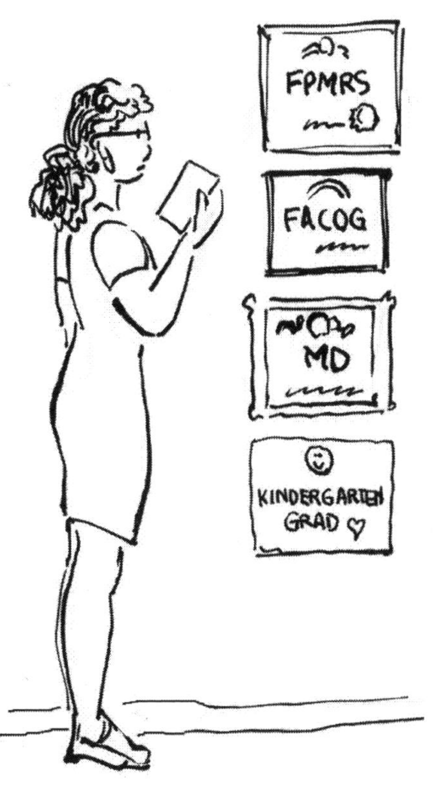

Surgical experience is the most important factor to consider in choosing a surgeon. You want to see someone who has done hundreds or even thousands of operations similar to the one you are considering – not just someone with good marketing. Ask him or her, how many surgeries like yours have they done? How often do they perform the surgery – every week, or just a few times a year?

You also want to see someone you like and trust. You have probably heard it said that some surgeons push patients into surgery. You want to make sure your surgeon is not “knife happy,” advising every woman who walks into his or her office that she needs an operation.

All surgeons make a living by doing surgery. That is fine, but some surgeons put their interest in making money ahead of what is best for you. Find a doctor you feel advises and treats you in the way they would a loved one of their own. That is what you deserve and what you should expect.

Choosing a Surgeon for Vaginal Tightening (Vaginoplasty/Perineoplasty)

For vaginal tightening, you should choose a gynecologist or urogynecologist who specializes in cosmetic gynecology, rather than a plastic surgeon who is doing cosmetic GYN surgery. All gynecologists and urogynecologists have delivered many babies during their post-medical school training. Their training in surgery focuses on the vagina and female pelvic organs.

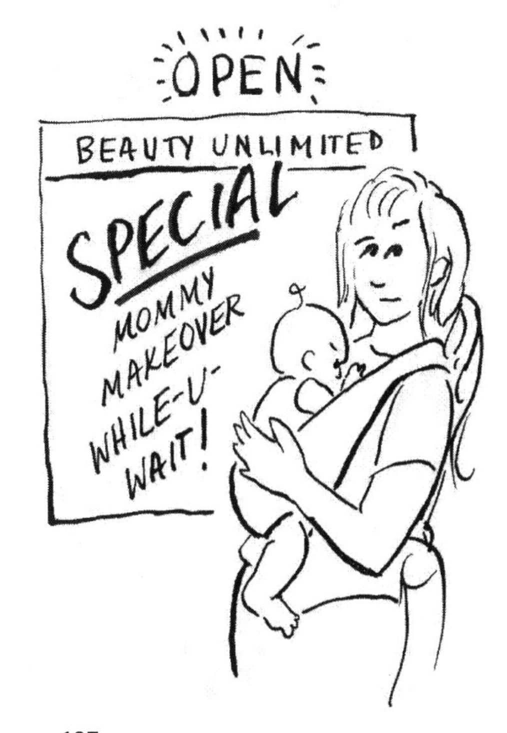

Plastic surgeons, on the other hand, deliver no babies during their training and do not operate on the vagina. Plastic surgeons do a lot of marketing. The "Mommy Makeover" is an example: Get your breasts fixed and abdomen flattened when you are finished having children! Since vaginoplasties have become more popular, there are a growing number of plastic surgeons advertising and offering vaginal tightening services to their patients. Plastic surgeons are not skilled at doing vaginal surgery. They have no in-depth experience or training.

Something to keep in mind when choosing a surgeon is this: Any woman who needs surgery for vaginal tightening also has pelvic organ prolapse to a greater or lesser degree. A woman who needs her vagina tightened always has a rectocele (prolapsed rectum). Other problems related to pelvic prolapse may exist as well.

Repairing pelvic prolapse of any kind is the area of surgical specialization of the urogynecologist, also known as a female pelvic reconstructive surgeon. This is a new subspecialty, formed in 2013, which combines expertise in both gynecology and urology. Because it is a new designation, you can still find general GYNs who are not FPMRS credentialled but who are skilled in surgical repair from many years of practice. The main consideration is this: If you need your vagina fixed, see someone with a background in gynecology, not plastic surgery.

This does not mean that any gynecologist or urogynecologist is a good choice - far from it. Most urogynecologists and gynecologists are not trained in cosmetic gynecology. Female genital plastic surgery (the other name for cosmetic gynecology) is a new field and there are no standard training programs or certifications. So again, the experience level of your doctor is the most important determining factor in choosing a surgeon.

You can easily gauge how well your doctor understands your problem by asking the doctor what kinds of symptoms other patients needing this surgery have had. If the doctor is not describing what you are experiencing, it's a signal the doctor hasn't treated enough patients. Also ask about other options for treatment in addition to surgery. There are always other options. Stay away from aggressive surgeons.

Choosing a Surgeon for Labiaplasty

In addition to gynecologists and urogynecologists who specialize in cosmetic gynecology, there are also plastic surgeons who do excellent work with labiaplasties. Since the labia are simply folds of skin which lie outside the body, a skilled and experienced cosmetic surgeon can alter this anatomy to improve physical appearance.

But once again, regardless of his or her specialty, your surgeon needs to focus on cosmetic gynecology. Don't see a plastic surgeon who just mentions this on their website along with ten other procedures. Most patients who see plastic surgeons are women. Some surgeons market for "all" cosmetic procedures patients are interested in.

In my practice, there are patients who come for a labiaplasty consultation - when all they really need is a simple gynecological medication to alleviate symptoms – not a procedure! A plastic surgeon will not offer you gynecology care.

PART 4

Having Surgery With Me

What To Expect With Surgery and How Your Life Might Change Afterward

In this section you will learn:

- What to expect at your consultation
- Before surgery
  - Medical evaluation before surgery
  - Common studies needed and pre-op surgery clearance
  - What to tell your loved ones or co-workers
- The day of surgery
  - Outpatient experience is fast
  - The day after surgery
  - How long to heal and when you can resume sex
- How surgery gives some women a fresh start in life
- The art of surgery
- A message to my patients - sharing my journey

Your Consultation and Surgery

More than half of our patients travel from out of state, many of them from thousands of miles away. But even if you live only an hour or two from my practice, it's easiest to start with a phone consultation before the in-person appointment. You can schedule a phone consultation with a message or e-mail to our office.

You will fill out a health questionnaire and take some private photos – photos of your privates – and send them to us before the phone consultation. (Your photos will be submitted to a secure medical site and saved as part of your protected medical records.)

I will call you at your scheduled time - give or take thirty minutes or so. We will have plenty of time to talk and have all your questions answered.

Most patients are soon comfortable sharing their problems and questions, even though the topic of discussion is not exactly cocktail party conversation. I feel compassion for your suffering, know how to help you, and have had these conversations thousands of times.

Based on our discussion and my review of your records and photos, I may recommend surgery as a good option for you. If you decide to proceed to the next step, Erica - my awesome surgery scheduler – will email or call you to get you scheduled for a physical exam.

At this point, many women who live far away will schedule their surgery for the day immediately following their physical exam, to avoid making two trips. Many women have been contemplating surgery for a long time: once they decide they are ready for surgery, they don't want to wait any longer.

Laboratory studies are required beforehand. Surgical clearance from your local doctor and an EKG is often recommended as well. I will answer all your questions during our initial phone conversation. But I will also put your contact data into my cell phone and send you my contact data. Before surgery, you may suddenly think of a question you

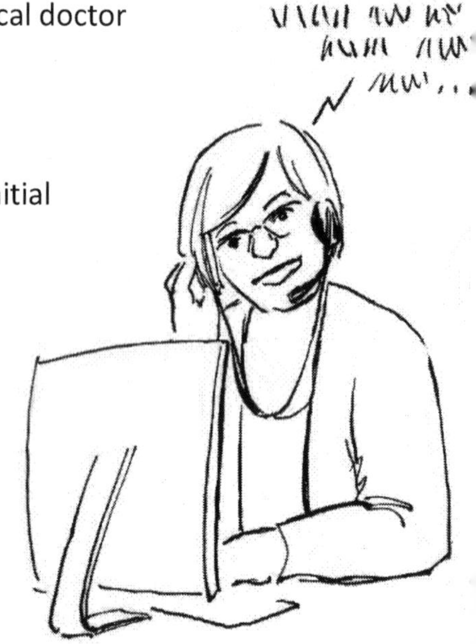

forgot to ask me, or afterward, additional questions may come to mind. You can text me any time before or after the surgery for any reason.

Medical Evaluation Before Surgery

Before you have any surgery, your overall health must be evaluated. Surgery has risks and requires healing. The healthier you are, the lower the risks and the faster the healing.

Most patients who want cosmetic gynecological surgery are healthy. It is a sign of health to be concerned both about your appearance, sexuality, and sexual relationships. An unhealthy person is generally not thinking about sex, the appearance of their genitals, physical attractiveness, how good they are in bed with their current partner – or about meeting someone new.

The medical evaluation boils down to: understanding the exact problem you want addressed, an evaluation of your medical history, your physical exam, confirming you have no undiagnosed medical problems, laboratory studies, other studies as needed, and at times asking another doctor to evaluate your health.

These are the basic categories of the medical evaluation:

1. “History of Present Illness” is just your description of what is bothering you and for how long. Other questions I may ask will help me understand whether your problem is isolated or part of something else. For example, if you complain about looseness in your vagina with sex, do you also have leakage?

2. “Your Past History” will include questions about past or present medical problems, any surgeries you have had, and your gynecological and obstetrical history. For example, how many pregnancies have you had and were there any problems? Do you have any gynecological problems, like a history of painful and/or heavy cycles?

Additional questions will ask you about pelvic pressure, pain with sex, bladder or stool leakage, and any history of abnormal Pap smears or sexual infections. I will also need to know how you prevent pregnancy, and are you planning more children?

3. “Medications and Allergies” is what it sounds like. Basic information, but important for me to know.

4. “Social History” includes questions to help me understand the kind of life you have, your support and

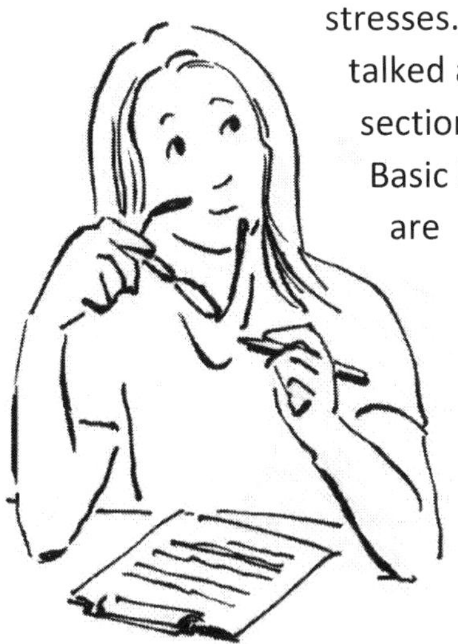

stresses. This is part of what I talked about in the first section of the book, "The 5 Basic Patient Types." You are not one-dimensional. Your healing journey is often about more than just your anatomy – sometimes it's about damage made worse by current life stresses or abusive past relationships. It is important to me as your surgeon to have a good idea what your life is like, so I can counsel you regarding having surgery in the first place – and also help guide you with the healing process.

I'll ask questions about what kind of work you do, who you live with, how many children you have and what their ages are. Also, I will ask about your current sexual partner, life stresses, any history with smoking (bad for healing, particularly with labiaplasties) or illicit drugs (also bad for healing – and for life in general).

5. A physical examination confirms that your complaint is related to something anatomical. As obvious as it sounds, only anatomical issues can be fixed with

surgery. When it comes to vaginal or labial surgery, if you can't easily understand the problem in my office, where you can look in a mirror while I do your physical exam, you don't need surgery. An exam also confirms there is nothing else physical that can cause problems with your surgery, and nothing else to address before your surgery or that might require additional testing.

6. "Review of Systems." It's important to communicate any other issues going on with the systems of your body, such as your digestive system, or your cardiovascular system, etc. This includes anything going on with your body. Changes in weight, bowels, and energy levels are common examples. Any other pains and discomforts, particularly in the chest or breathing or abdomen or pelvis. Any skin lesions or lumps you have noticed. It's better to share details before you have surgery because sometimes other problems are found that require more immediate action.

7. Laboratory studies confirm that you are healthy and don't have other problems that first need to be addressed. A recent Pap smear is needed before any GYN surgery. (A Pap smear is a scraping of your cervix or vagina to screen for cancer or precancer lesions.)

Blood work should include a Complete Blood Count (CBC) to make sure your blood is normal, and a test called a PT/PTT to evaluate for abnormal bleeding. You'll also need to be evaluated for infections with a cervical swab for chlamydia and gonorrhea. These infections, when present in your vagina, can cause serious infection after surgery if they are not treated. Evaluation also includes blood work to test for hepatitis, syphilis, and HIV. A test for prediabetes or diabetes, called a hemoglobin A 1c, is a good idea as well.

Common Studies Sometimes Needed Before Surgery

A pelvic ultrasound is commonly performed. This is to look at your internal anatomy to make certain all is normal. Don't have cosmetic and elective gynecological surgery without good evaluation for common problems that can be treated at the same time.

A bladder study or urodynamics is done if you have issues with bladder leakage.

Anorectal Manometry (ARM) is done if you have stool leakage, constipation or certain bowel issues.

An EKG is sometimes recommended to evaluate the electrical conduction of your heart.

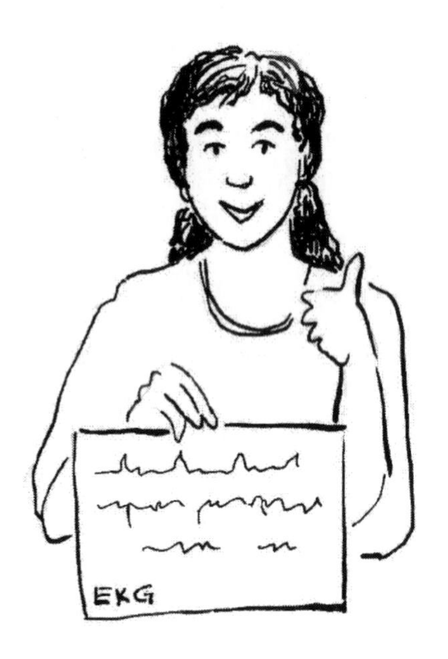

Preoperative Surgical Clearance

If you have any medical risk factors, including age or weight, evaluation before surgery by your internist or cardiologist may be recommended to confirm you are healthy enough to have surgery. An EKG will usually be performed, and at times an Echocardiogram – or an ultrasound of your heart.

What to Tell Loved Ones or Coworkers About Your Plans

Some patients are comfortable screaming from the rooftops, "My vagina is too loose, and I want it fixed!" Others want to keep their personal business personal.

If you want to protect your privacy from loved ones and coworkers, simply tell them you are having bladder leakage fixed, or pelvic organ prolapse from childbirth repaired, or simply that you have a hernia that needs an operation.

It is not uncommon for some patients to arrive with travel companions who don't know what they are having done. My recommendation is to keep this person out of our office. But if you want them to accompany you at certain times during your care, simply tell me, so I can write a private note on your chart. We are very discreet.

Your First Visit – for Patients Arriving After a Phone Consult

At your first office visit, a physical examination will be performed. A hand mirror will be used to help you see and understand your anatomy. Photographs will be taken both before and after surgery. (Again, photos are part of your protected medical records.)

Sometimes other studies are ordered, such as an ultrasound or bladder study. My awesome assistant Kami and I will make sure you feel comfortable and that everything goes smoothly.

You will receive prescriptions for pain medications before you leave. Fill these that evening so they are ready after surgery. Buy some stool softeners such as Colace to take for three weeks or longer after the surgery. Get some plastic bottles of water to place in the freezer as a convenient way to ice your bottom after surgery. Buy some comfort food, too, so your recovery is - well, more comfortable.

You can eat and drink whatever you want the evening before surgery. Erica and Kami will give you a list of nice restaurants nearby as well as some local attractions. Come a few days before your surgery if you want to

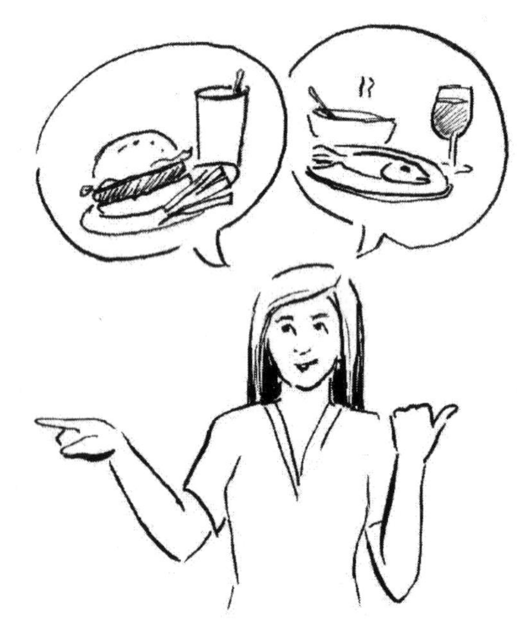

sight-see. Do not plan to sight-see after surgery when you need to be resting.

Stop eating or drinking eight hours before your surgery is scheduled.

The Day of the Surgery

You will arrive about an hour before your surgery is scheduled.

You will meet our nurse anesthetist, who will place an IV into your arm. You also will have topical numbing cream placed on your genitals by a medical assistant. You will be escorted to our operating room where you will change.

My excellent surgical team, Maricarmen and Monica, will prepare you for surgery. This includes cleaning the surgical area and covering you with sterile drapes. Once everything is set, you will receive some light sedation and additional numbing medication. The surgery will begin. You will not feel a thing. We will be done before you know it.

Once you are back in your recovery room, we will place some ice on your bottom and give you some water and crackers. You will be ready to leave in about thirty minutes.

Take some pain medication when you get back to your hotel, even if it doesn't hurt. The pain increases as the numbing medication wears off in two or three hours. Take a nap. You can resume your normal diet. Take your stool softeners, too.

If you just had a labiaplasty, you will feel fine. Make sure you use ice and take it slowly. Excessive activity can cause bleeding because the labia on the outside of the body can become irritated.

Vaginoplasties hurt more. The most common complaint after surgery is the feeling you need to have a bowel movement. This is the sensation of "rectal pressure." A tighter vagina puts pressure on your rectum, as does packing inside your vagina. Surgical packing is 2-inch-wide cotton dressing, 18 to 24 inches long. It is usually removed the following day.

The Day After Surgery

To help you rest, Kami or Maricarmen will come to your hotel room the next morning for the post-op check-up so you do not have to return to the office. They will check your incisions, take out your packing, and answer all your questions.

You should plan to rest all day and catch up on your beauty sleep. Most patients can be driven home the day after surgery. But if you take a flight, we recommend your return flight be at least two or three days after the surgery.

Listen to your body.

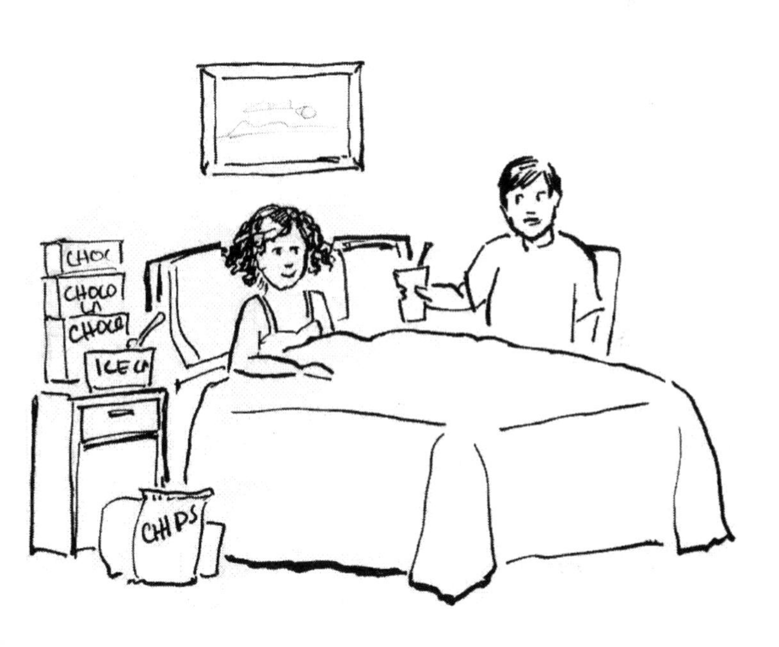

The First Week After Surgery

The first three to seven days are when you experience the most discomfort. For vaginoplasty surgery, the rectal pressure is the worst feeling. This will be better before the week is out. But constipation can occur, which exacerbates and confuses the issue. Constipation occurs because of the narcotic pain medication and decreased activity. Make sure you drink plenty of water and take stool softeners. Once you are walking, you will have a bowel movement. If you have difficulty, I may advise an enema. Showers and baths are fine after a vaginoplasty – but if you had a labiaplasty, just do showers.

The discomfort with labiaplasty surgery is only about three days. But you will have significant swelling which can last more than a month. It is essential you ice yourself as much as you can tolerate that first week. Don't sit in a tub the first week as this can loosen the sutures. Showers are fine.

The First Two Months After Surgery

You will feel better each week. Unless you have a physically demanding job, you can return to work after a week or so of rest. You can text me questions as they come up. Many patients text me photos to show areas of concern. Swelling normally occurs during the healing process. Most of the time, any irregularity is just part of the normal healing process. Your final appearance can take as long as three to six months to resolve.

If you notice a yellow discharge that has an odor, you may need to take a week of antibiotics. Almost half of patients experience this. The dissolving sutures can cause an overgrowth of bacteria. Often, I send you home with a prescription in case this happens. Text me and I will direct your care.

I will typically see you six to eight weeks after surgery before you become sexually active. I will see you earlier if there are any issues.

Returning to Sexual Activity

Wait at least eight weeks before resuming sexual intercourse. Some women may take longer. Everyone heals at a different pace. An easy way to tell if you are ready is to use your thumb to press down on the back of your vagina. If you hurt, you are not ready. Listen to your body. For labiaplasties, pinch your labia with your thumb and index finger. If you hurt, you are not ready. Make sense?

Orgasm is an important part of health and happiness. After a vaginoplasty, clitoral orgasm without vaginal penetration is fine, once your desire returns. Because

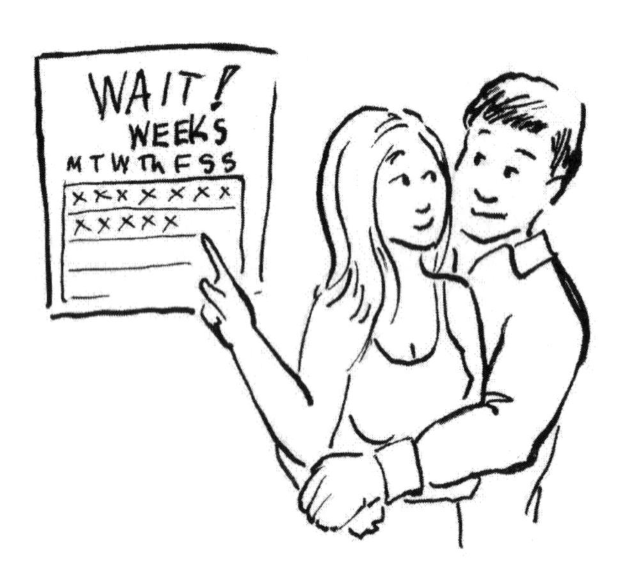

the clitoral area was not involved with the surgery, this is completely safe.

With labiaplasty, however, you will need to wait at least three weeks for clitoral orgasm. The labia are attached to the skin that covers the clitoris, so massaging this area can disrupt the sutures. After three weeks - before you attempt clitoral orgasm - make sure the labia are not tender or significantly swollen. At that point, you should be ok.

Take it slowly. Once you initiate sexual intercourse, a female dominant position (the woman on top) helps you control depth and rate of penetration. Lubrication is fine to use. You may experience pain or even mild bleeding at first. Don't worry. Your new and improved body will become used to sexual intercourse in time. If the tightness or pain continues for more than two months, you may need medication, physical therapy, or vaginal dilators. If the tightness is not as much as you desire, physical therapy with muscle strengthening is indicated.

Keep me informed about how everything is going, and I will advise you what needs to be done.

Surgery Can Give a Fresh Start

For many women, the decision to have reconstructive gynecological surgery is an intense period of self-reflection. One patient commented, "It's almost like restoring physical virginity and considering very seriously who is worthy of such an intimate act, makes the stakes higher. Connecting sex to both body and soul makes it seem exactly like it should be."

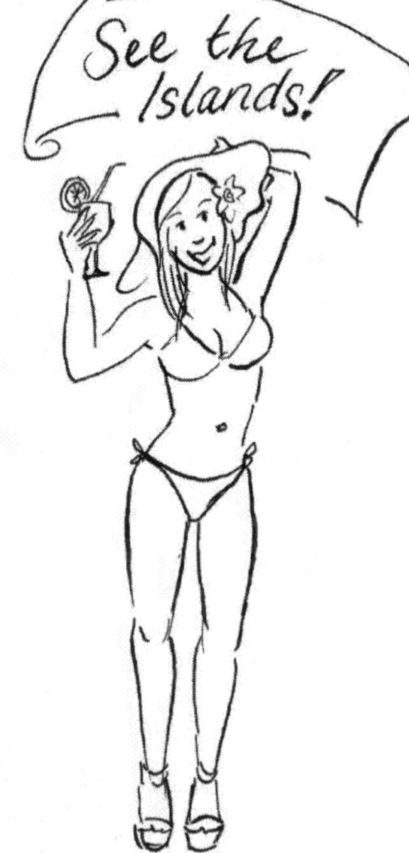

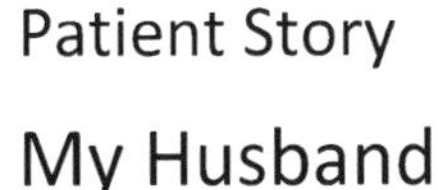

Patient Story

My Husband Left Me to Become a Woman

"My husband was a closet homosexual. I couldn't believe it when I found out. He was having homosexual affairs for years and dressing like a woman. He wasn't even apologetic when I finally caught him. We got divorced, but not before he gave me genital warts. I guess it could have been worse.

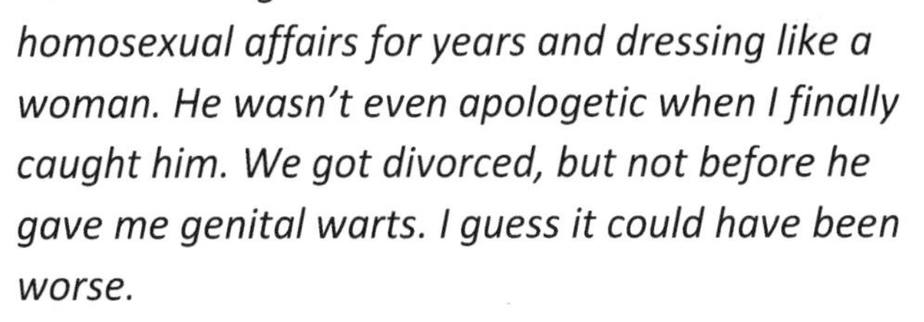

Our kids were still teenagers and so hurt and confused. My ex brought his gay lover to school events right away - like that was helpful. It was a hard time. I went through a lot of bottles of wine back then!

I gave up on sex for a long time. I gave up on a lot of things. But after my kids were grown, I wanted to do something for myself. I lost weight and had Dr. Litrel fix all my lady parts. Things were messed up down there and lots of times I wondered if there wasn't something wrong with me that caused all this. I knew it wasn't really me, of course, but I couldn't get away from the feeling that my marriage fell apart because I wasn't sexy enough.

I've finally started dating again. I actually feel good about myself! I realize now none of this was my fault or about me. I got unlucky, but God blessed me with three beautiful children – and now a whole new life!"

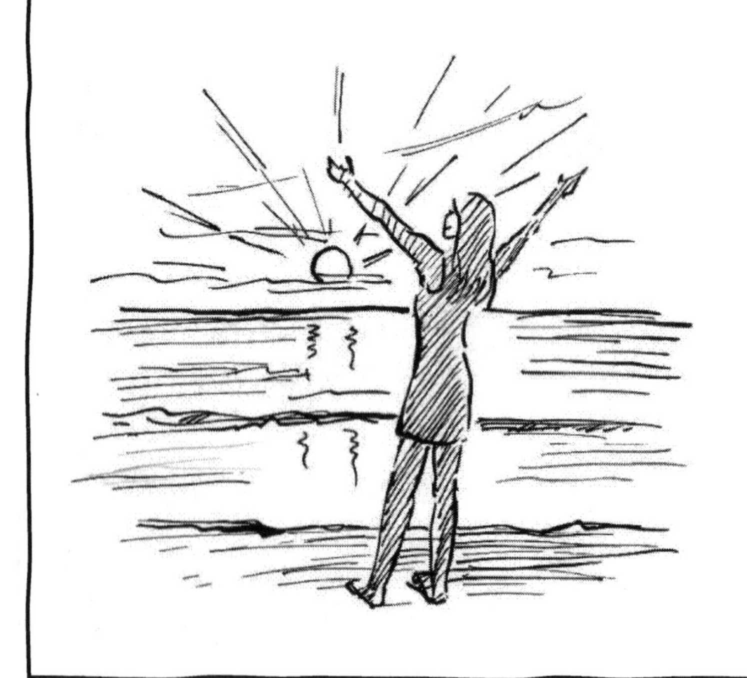

The Art of Surgery

The summer of my junior year in college, I befriended an elderly artist. I was an EMT (emergency medical technician) for a private ambulance company, and I met Maria one evening when I took her from her nursing home to her doctor's office. Unlike the typical sterile bedroom of every nursing home I saw, Maria's room was full of books and paintings and sculptures. Maria was an artist, an intellectual who spoke six languages and studied deeply many subjects.

Maria became a dear friend, and before her passing just three years later, an important life mentor for me.

I want to share the three foundational lessons Maria taught me. The first two I have followed diligently throughout my life. The third has taken me longer to understand, and I am only now putting it into words.

Maria first gave me life advice about ambition. As a young man, I was hungry for success and recognition. I imagined I would become an important professor of medicine at a prestigious university, traveling around the world, lecturing and teaching and pontificating. Maria suffered as a refugee during World War II. She saw many die - and almost died herself several times. Her advice to me was patient, loving and simple.

Avoid the Limelight and Stay Away from the Fuss.

"Avoid the limelight. Raise your family away from the fuss. Live in a small town. Ann can paint (my then fiancé and now wife is an artist, too). You can be a doctor. Take care of your patients. Spend time with your children. You will be happy."

I have practiced in a small town north of Atlanta for 25 years. My goal is to practice another 25.

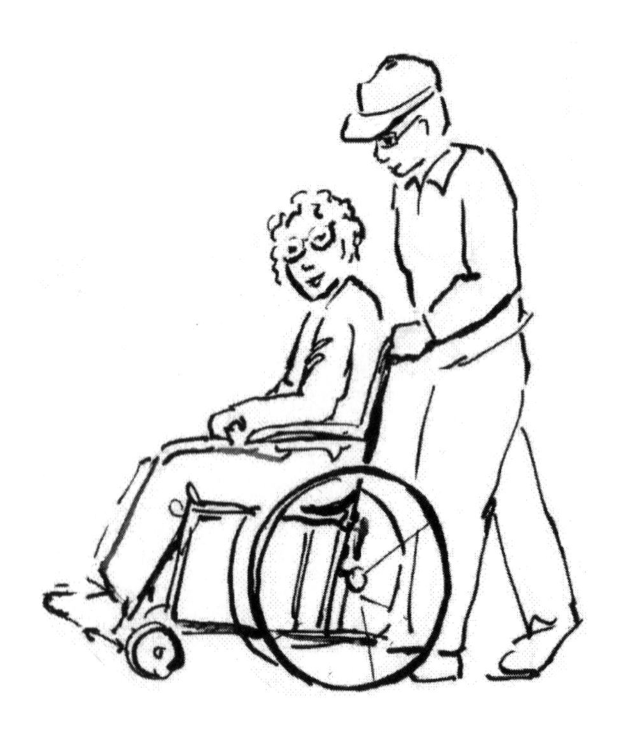

Be Honest. Don't Pretend.

The other advice Maria gave me was about intellectual honesty. Although I was a busy college student, Maria gave me many reading assignments to further my education. They encompassed many subjects ranging widely from art history, to Gnostic gospels, to quantum physics. The one time Maria chastised me in a letter was because I failed to look up a word I did not know, and thus had glossed over a key concept she wanted me to understand. "Never pretend to know something you don't," was her admonition. "Pay attention to the meaning of each word." It was the only time Maria had become impatient with me.

The take home message for me has been this: Intellectual honesty is important. You must know what you know, and also know what you don't know. All this sounds obvious, but it bears mentioning simply because it is a gross misconception that doctors have the answers. Many doctors hide behind a complicated vocabulary that is nothing more than an affectation of understanding. I have studied medicine all my adult life, and I assure you that doctors do not know the most basic things about life: Why do we need sleep? Or why do we age? Or even, exactly how does the body heal? And that's just biology.

We know even less about the more important questions in life – like, where do we come from, what is the purpose of life, how do we live in order to be happy and fulfilled, and where do we go when our bodies die? Existential questions may seem out of place in a book about surgery, but these questions are fundamental to our life journey and our true health.

We are not human beings having spiritual problems. We are spiritual beings having human problems.

My understanding of my task as a healer and surgeon is this: Listen, observe, and act with a humble, loving heart. When I serve my patient and God to the best of my ability, I am blessed to witness the miracle and joy of God's healing grace.

Art Is Simply Taking Away What Doesn't Belong.

The third thing Maria taught me was about Art. "Being a sculptress is easy," she told me one day with a laugh. "All you do is take away what does not belong. Simple!"

I was not sure what she meant. Her statement seemed either totally profound - or total BS.

But thirty years later, I think I now understand Maria's lesson. Surgery is both an art and a science. When I was a young doctor, surgery was more science than art. But now after decades of practice, it has come to be more art than science. Science is about thinking and understanding. Art is about feeling and knowing.

Instead of stone or clay, the artistic medium of the surgeon is the human body. The surgeon's job is simply to take away what does not belong.

I have examined over a hundred thousand women, of all ages, with all sorts of problems or no problems at all. I have delivered thousands of babies. I have performed thousands of surgeries. There is a way a woman looks before she is sexually active, before and after she has children, and a way she looks after she experiences the changes that come with aging and normal health challenges. It is not possible to surgically repair your body so it is exactly as it was when you were eighteen years old. But that remains the esthetic and reconstructive surgical goal.

It seems to me the essence of a woman's beauty emanates from the sacrifices she endures in creating new life. There may be no human experience which rivals the challenge and suffering of growing another human being inside the body, followed by the loving and unrelenting work of years of motherhood. And while the miracle of pregnancy endows every mother with beauty of the spirit, childbirth ironically mounts a full assault on beauty of the body, employing a small battering ram in the form of the baby's head.

Surgery of female genitalia has a simple goal: Repair the damage, return your anatomy to the way it was. Take away what doesn't belong, so the beauty can shine out.

After performing a hundred thousand gynecological exams, I finally understand what Maria said about sculpting so many years ago –

"It's simple."

The Journey

Love, Beauty and Spirituality

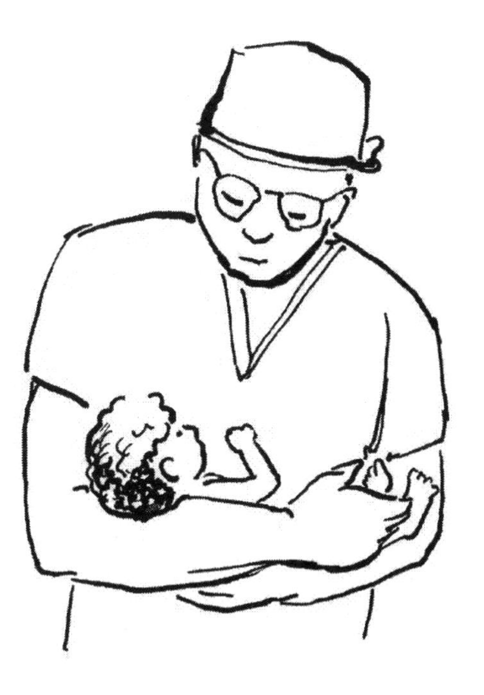

I have known I wanted to be a doctor since I was seven years old. I had cut my leg badly, and a stranger in a white coat with a reassuring smile sutured the laceration. As I watched him repair my body, the terror in my heart transformed alchemically to awe. It became my dream to one day help someone as frightened as I was, someone who really needed me.

I delivered my first baby as a third-year medical student.

It was just before dawn, and I was at the hospital on my first overnight call as a third-year student. It took over an hour for the nineteen-year old mother to push her baby out. I watched as her baby's head emerged, and then retracted. The screams of the young woman echoed against the blue green tiles of the operating room. Diarrhea squirted from her swollen anus. Finally, with a scream of agony, the young mother, her vagina and vulva tearing, pushed her baby's head out.

Guided by the Intern, I suctioned the baby's mouth and nostrils and then delivered the baby. It was a girl. Terrified of dropping her, I clutched her tiny form in both arms as the intern clamped and cut the umbilical cord for me.

And within moments, I understood it was my destiny to be an obstetrician and gynecologist.

In the ten seconds it took for me to place the baby on the warmer, I felt myself lifted out of my body. No longer was I walking on the tiled floor, my body limited to the delivery room on the 13th floor of Atlanta's Grady Memorial Hospital – I was floating, hyper-aware of everything around me, and connected to something far greater. I put the baby down and turned back to the young mother to deliver the placenta and assist the Intern with the surgical repair.

The feeling of unbearable spiritual elation stayed with me for almost a full minute. And as I processed the emotion, I thought to myself, "Holy shit – I think I am supposed to become an OB-GYN!"

No one was more surprised than I was.

My opinion about obstetrics and gynecology had been formed ten years earlier, when I had asked my high school girlfriend how her first gynecology appointment went. She simply grimaced and shook her head, her blue eyes welling with tears. I became angry. On that day I was certain of one thing: if I ever became a doctor, it would never be a specialty that made young women cry.

God has a sense of humor.

Women and Men

I am grateful to God for the opportunity to care for women. In caring for women, I have come to believe that women have more difficult lives than we men do. A woman is biologically and spiritually hardwired to sustain the difficulties of pregnancy, birth, and motherhood. A woman is the vessel through which God creates new life.

Men and women appear to me to remain different in a number of fundamental ways. Men participate in the creation of life – but only through a woman's body. I sometimes wonder if there is an inherited biological selflessness of women – giving life to others – along with a biological selfishness to men – taking from others.

Women go around wondering about the needs of others and how they can help. Many men seem to go around wondering what they want, and what they must to do to get it.

Sex, too, is different for women and men. Intimacy and love matter more for women, the demand for physical gratification matters less. I am not saying that men do not want intimacy and love, or that women do not want mind-blowing orgasms. But when it comes to sexual intercourse, the genders have different biological purposes.

For men, ejaculation is the goal and the end.

For women, a man's ejaculation is only the beginning.

Put another way, a man can spend ten minutes with sex and then fall asleep. A woman can spend nine months of misery, ending in an agonizing delivery – and then suffer another eighteen years of motherhood to boot.

Sex is important and should be enjoyed. But true intimacy with another requires love and commitment, not just the physical pleasure of sexual intercourse.

Learning to Love

A woman's genitalia are the part of her body for receiving and giving sexual pleasure – and of course, the passageway for new life. But when the genitalia are damaged, they often affect not just a woman's sex life, but also her ability to love herself.

When you do not feel good about yourself or love yourself enough, you cannot love others as much as you want. This is a spiritual truth.

The bodily sacrifices of womanhood are why patients come to me for medical care and corrective surgery. Surgery is about the body, of course.

But when it comes to sex and relationships, the body forms just part of the equation. Over the years, women have come to this office and confided the source of their pain and unhappiness. Most times, a woman's full health – physical and emotional - has to do with her relationships with others and the never-ending challenge of self-love.

We are not human beings having spiritual problems. We are spiritual beings having human problems.

My goal is to help my patients find true healing. Surgical correction to beautify and reconstruct a woman's genitalia can be a n important part of the healing process, a step on the road to the physical and spiritual health every woman deserves.

The one thing that can improve with the years of our life is our ability to love – love ourselves, others, and God. And that of course, is the purpose of life.

Many blessings on your healing journey.

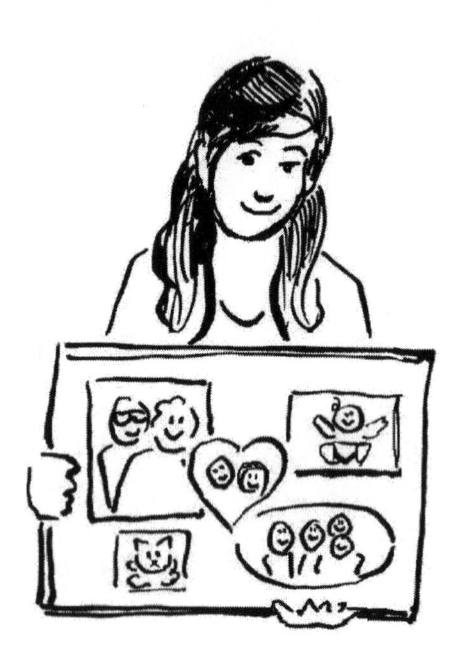

About the Author

Dr. Michael Litrel

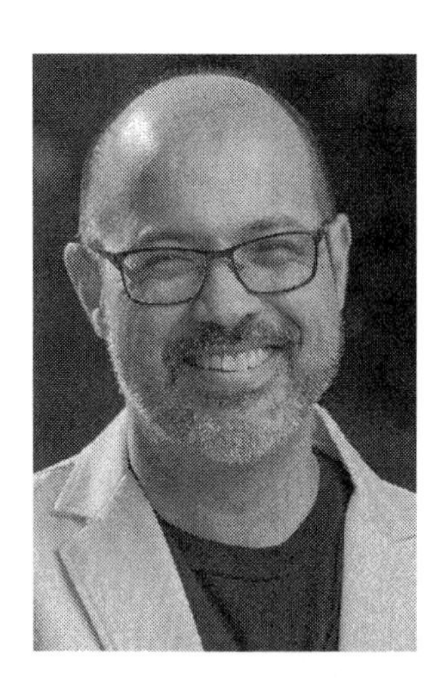

Is a urogynecological and female reconstructive cosmetic surgeon, double board-certified in Female Pelvic Medicine and Reconstructive Surgery (FPMRS) and in Obstetrics and Gynecology. For over twenty years, Dr. Litrel delivered the babies of thousands of women in his community, witnessing firsthand the effects of childbirth on his patients' anatomy and sexual function. As a urogynecologist, Dr. Litrel has built on that experience to develop new techniques in female genital cosmetic and reconstructive surgery, repairing the natural anatomy of women to restore sexual and functional pelvic anatomy. His patients include thousands of women who travel from every state and multiple countries to experience his surgical expertise and his trademark approach to helping women with their surgery, and for many, the healing journey of their life. Read his patients' reviews on www.RealSelf.com

Reading Group Questions and Topics for Discussion

1. The journey of healing is a primary theme in "Sex, Your Body and Your Relationships." Were you surprised to see women seeking healing through GYN surgery?

When you are hurting or have suffered loss, what kinds of things help you get back on track – whether exercise, travel, or little things like a new outfit or a massage? Do you think plastic surgery or cosmetic GYN has a place there for some?

2. The stories of several women throughout the book illustrate the idea that taking care of yourself is difficult. On page 21, Tessa, suffering from pelvic prolapse, is described as having a guilty feeling that she should accept her body the way it is. On page 59, we hear the story of a woman who is always taking care of others - her kids and her mother - feeling selfish for wanting to improve her sex life. Do you think women have a problem prioritizing their needs against the needs of others? What feelings or guidelines do you use to decide on your priorities regarding personal needs versus those of marriage, family, or career?

3. There are examples of women having surgery so they can get a clean start in life or in their relationships. On page 30, a woman describes wanting to feel attractive and fixed after a divorce. On page 35, a woman suffering from childhood sexual abuse chooses vaginoplasty to feel clean again for her husband. Do you think it's possible to get a clean start by having surgery on the body? In what other ways have you seen women struggle with getting a clean start in their relationships or in life?

4. One reason for a woman choosing natural childbirth is named on page 55 as: "Some women need to feel it all." What are the reasons you would recommend, or not recommend, natural childbirth?

Beginning on page 63, a brief history of changes in obstetrical practices over the past half century is given. Were you surprised by any part of this explanation of damage to a woman's anatomy from natural childbirth?

Do you think the latest trends in medicine and science are ever an improvement over natural/holistic paths? Can you think of a time when trusted sources failed you, or when they were better/different from the experts?

5. The book contains several statements about men and women and how they differ. In the section

“Women and Men” beginning on page 167, we read that women have “an inherited biological selflessness,” that they “go around wondering about the needs of others and how they can help,” and that “intimacy and love matter more for women, the demand for gratification matters less [than for men].” How do the statements made in this section compare with your opinions about sex or gender?

6. Starting on page 159, Dr. Litrel tells the story of Maria, an older female mentor who taught him important life lessons which shaped his later decisions. Have you ever had a mentor, and if so, what were the lessons they taught you?

One of Maria’s lessons was “Be honest. Don’t Pretend.” On page 161, the author asserts that “many doctors hide behind a complicated vocabulary that is nothing more than an affectation of understanding.” What does that mean? Have you ever been surprised by an experience with a doctor or another “expert” – and if yes, in a positive or negative way?

7. The idea of “restoring virginity”’ and the reasons for doing it in some cultures are described beginning on page 113. What did you think of the young woman who is typically found in this situation? Is it okay to help someone even if you don’t agree with their

culture or beliefs? When, if ever, do you “draw the line”? Can you think of an incident where you or someone else was asked to help someone who had made choices that seemed bad or were difficult to agree with? How did that influence the desire or decision to help?

8. Some of the GYN surgery described in the book is reconstructive and some is considered cosmetic. What societal forces do you think are causing the field of cosmetic GYN to be growing? Do you believe the new specialty is beneficial for women, that it represents more choice and freedom, or do you consider it one more societal pressure?

What were your opinions before reading the book, if any, and were they changed by the book?

If you enjoyed this book,
you may enjoy these books, also by Dr. Litrel:

Family – A MisMatch Made In Heaven: Surviving True Love, Children, and Other Blessings In Disguise

The fairy tale begins when we fall in love. But what happens in "happily ever after?"

Dr. Litrel shares his experiences as a husband and father, trading stories with his artist wife Ann in this "he said-she said" book about family. They humorously share often opposite viewpoints on parenting with honesty and laugh-out-loud humor, showing how conflict, everyday gripes and family struggles can form a perfect recipe for learning how to love. Their stories about marriage and family provide the ultimate reassurance: It's okay to be human.

The Eyes Don't See – What Patients Can Teach Doctors About Medicine: Lessons In the Power of Miracles and Love

What can patients teach doctors about medicine?

That science, technology, pills and training only go so far. Real healing begins with faith. Dr. Litrel tells the dramatic and inspirational accounts of the patients he met in inner city Atlanta's famous Grady Hospital. These true stories of miracles in the operating room will restore your belief in the power of love and faith to change and save lives, showing that miracles do happen, every day.

Making the Faith/Health Connection –
A Companion Bible Study for <u>The Eyes Don't See</u>
Student Study Book and Teacher's Guide versions

A companion Bible study by Elizabeth Wallace, PhD, this 12-week series explores the connection between faith and health. Building on the miracle stories of Dr. Litrel's book *The Eyes Don't See,* each story is paired with relevant Bible study and discussion questions, bringing to life the 2,000-year-old wisdom shared by the most famous Healer of all. A new look at the subject of faith, health and miracles, illuminated in the modern day setting of an inner city hospital.

This 12-week series is suitable for self-guided reading as well as small group study. Complete Teacher's Guide also available.

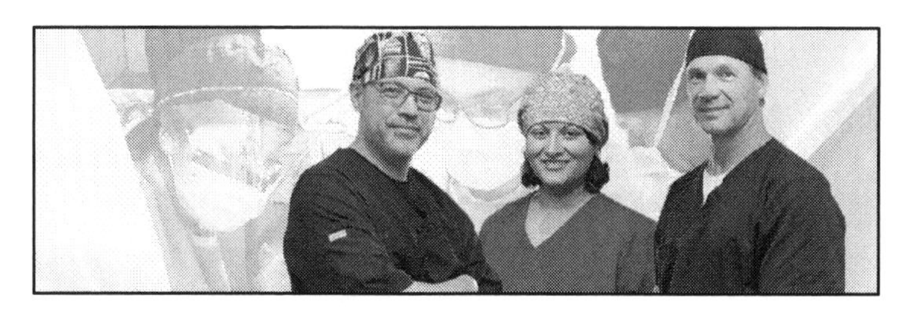

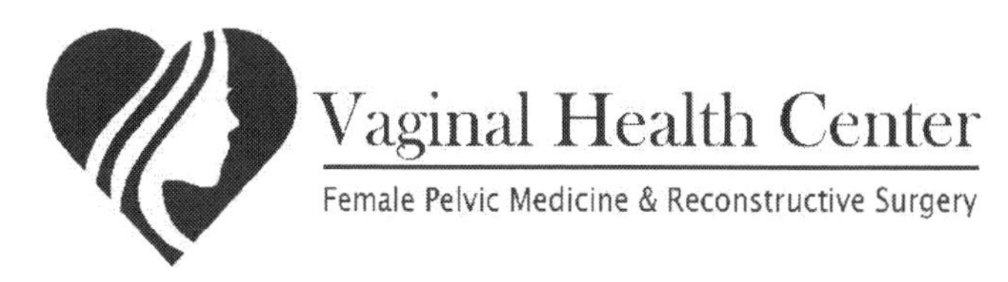
Vaginal Health Center
Female Pelvic Medicine & Reconstructive Surgery

With their training and years of experience, they have a further and complete understanding of a women's anatomy and the changes that occur after childbirth. Female Pelvic Medicine and Reconstructive Surgery specialists address both the internal and external changes to the vagina due to age or childbirth.

The team at Vaginal Health Center has a national reputation of excellence in providing expert care to women from the around the country. Women who take an active role in their vaginal health find that they are not alone and have a variety of options for restoring their quality of life. Our physicians help women navigate the path to healthy relationships, wellness, and restoration.

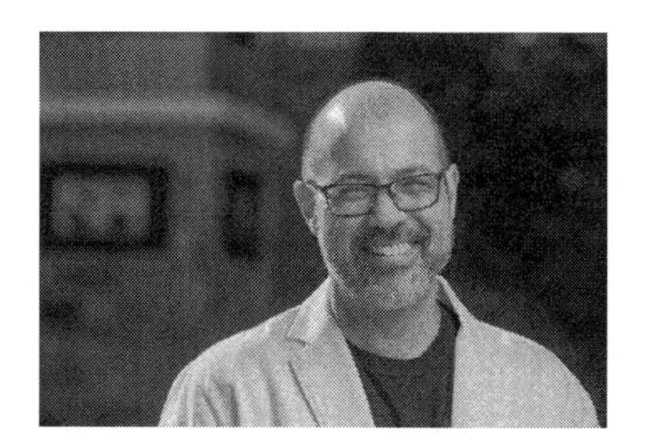

Michael Litrel, MD, FACOG, FPMRS
is a nationally recognized female pelvic reconstructive cosmetic surgeon and urogynecologist, double board-certified in the subspecialty Female Pelvic Medicine and Reconstructive Surgery and in Obstetrics and Gynecology. As an educator, author, and award-winning 'Top Doctor', Dr. Litrel helps women from across the country who seek expert help in this highly specialized field of surgical expertise.

"Women suffer and sacrifice themselves in incredible and loving ways for others. Using my surgical skills to restore their bodies from childbirth damage has been an honor and blessing, and I'm grateful every day for the opportunity to care for and help my patients."

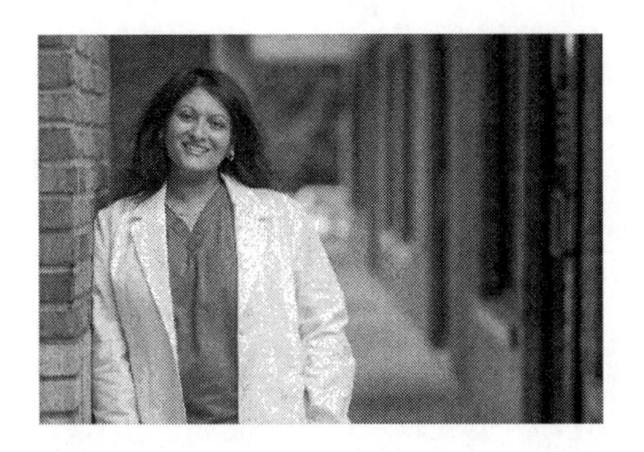

Peahen Gandhi, MD, FACOG, FPMRS is a urogynecological and female pelvic reconstructive surgeon, double board-certified in the subspecialty Female Pelvic Medicine and Reconstructive Surgery and in Obstetrics and Gynecology. As an award winning 'Top Doctor' and surgeon, she continues to help thousands of women obtain their optimal health.

"A good doctor should listen a lot and get the whole story, not just one simple complaint. I like the quote by Shakti Gawain, 'Our bodies communicate to us clearly and specifically, if we are willing to listen to them'. I like to think that I genuinely care and listen to my patients' needs, and that helps guide my recommendations."

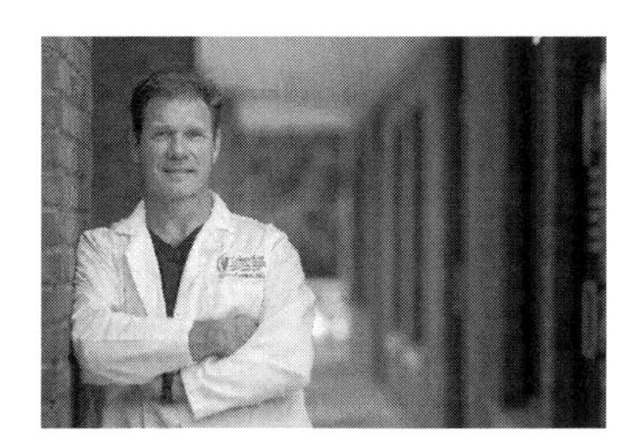

James Haley, MD, FACOG, FPMRS is a urogynecologist and advanced female pelvic reconstructive surgeon, double board-certified in the subspecialty Female Pelvic Medicine and Reconstructive Surgery and in Obstetrics and Gynecology. As an award-winning top surgeon, he has helped thousands of women who seek his expertise.

"I love a challenge, so I thrive in situations when a woman comes to me with a complex medical problem. I will do everything in my power to find a solution. The more complicated the problem, the more I excel. I have made it my lifelong goal to help women achieve optimal health."

Made in the USA
Monee, IL
24 September 2021

78113064R00107